'SEx Libris

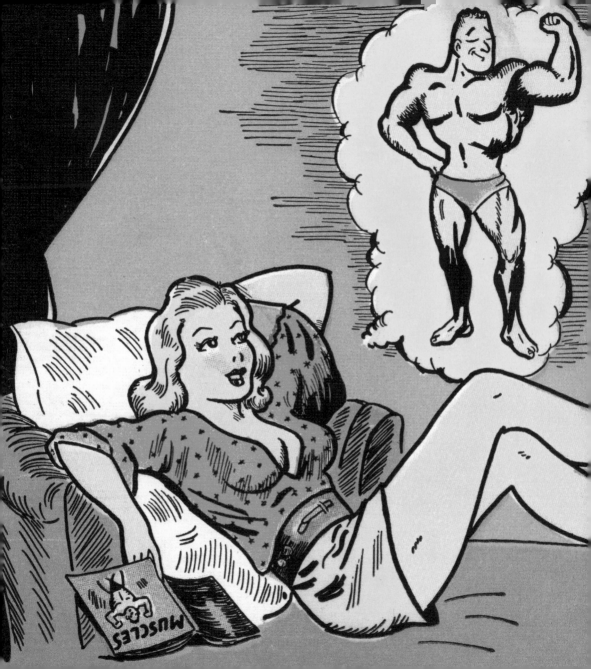

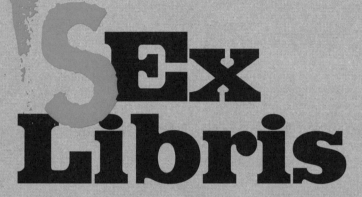

SEx Libris

A BOOK ABOUT WHAT EVERYONE THINKS THEY KNOW

FOREWORD BY **JAMIE BUFALINO**
(TIME OUT NEW YORK'S SEXPERT COLUMNIST)

EDITED BY **CHRISTOPHER MEASOM**

DESIGNED BY **TIMOTHY SHANER**

Published in 2007 by Welcome Books
An imprint of Welcome Enterprises, Inc.
6 West 18th Street, New York, NY 10011
Tel: 212-989-3200; Fax: 212-989-3205
www.welcomebooks.com

Publisher: Lena Tabori
Project Director: Alice Wong   Project Assistant: Kara Mason

Library of Congress Cataloging-in-Publication Data

Sex libris : the book about what everyone thinks they know / edited by
Christopher Measom; designed by Timothy Shaner. — 1st ed.
    p. cm.
  ISBN 978-1-59962-024-4 (alk. paper)
1. Sex. 2. Sex—Humor. 3. Sex (Psychology) 4. Sex in literature.
I. Measom, Christopher.
  HQ21.S47178 2007
  306.77--dc22   2007013470

ISBN 978-1-59962-024-4

Printed in Singapore

FIRST EDITION
1 3 5 7 9 10 8 6 4 2

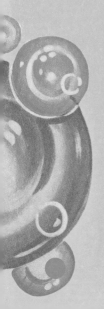
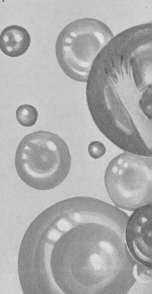

CONTENTS

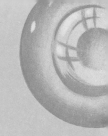

CONTENTS

CONTENTS

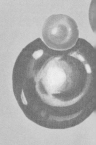

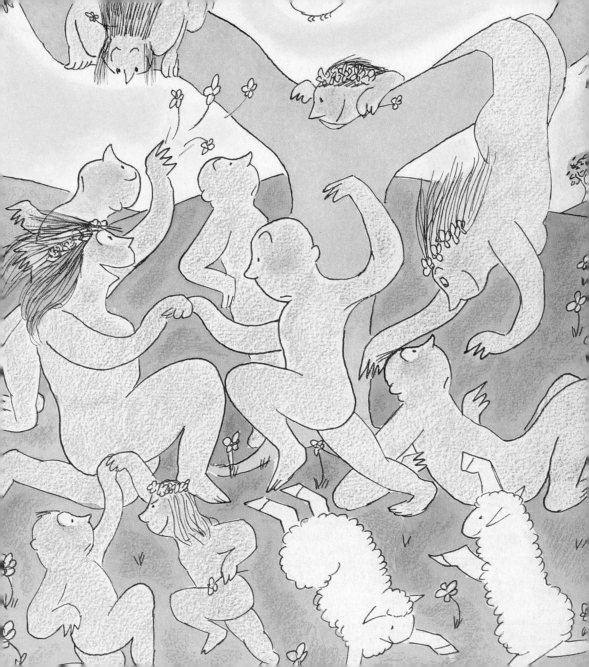

FOREWORD

Picture this: Two tall, leafy oak trees tower over a suburban backyard. A white rope hammock connects the trees, looking like a strand of spit caught between two sloppy kissers who just came up for air. It's a scorching summer day, and an overheated couple decide to make good use of the hammock. He takes off all his clothes and stretches out facedown, so that his manhood dangles through one of the hammock's square holes. She takes off all her clothes and lies on the grass under the hammock. Fellatio ensues.

Now, none of this happened to me, you understand. But I still consider the dangling hammock action to be the moment of my sexual awakening. I was eleven or twelve or thirteen, or whatever that age is when a boy's hormones kick in and suddenly almost every bit of alone time is spent with his hand in his underpants. Mind you, no one had taught me to put my hands in my underpants; the idea came to

me all on its own, much like, I imagine, the way a
more devout boy might get the notion to join the
priesthood: It was a calling from the universe. It
was the universe that nudged me to snoop around
my parents' bedroom. It was the universe that led to
me to the cubbyhole in their walk-in closet. It was
the universe that placed a lowbrow sex manual in
that cubbyhole (it was the universe, I tell you, not
my mom, good God, not my mom). It was the universe that convinced me there would be much fun
to be had should I abscond with this lowbrow sex
manual, spend a few hours leafing through it in the
privacy of my bedroom, and perhaps happen upon
a page containing an extremely inventive use for a
hammock. Yes, the universe brought me to that
family, that cubbyhole, that book, that page, but it
was ultimately the hammock couple who unleashed
the neural-hormonal-biomechanical chain of events
that ended with my hand thrust into my underpants,
and my eyes finally opened to the explosive world
of sexuality.

I am, therefore, a living, breathing, underpants-spunking testament to the joy that can be wrought from a book about sex. And now you hold in your hands the chance to have a sexual awakening (one in a long line, no doubt) of your own. Who knows what erotic word or suggestive photo or naughty illustration contained in these pages will suddenly spark the fires in you: Japanese warriors, maybe, phone sex, Moorish harems, ponygirls, or perhaps a thrusting thrashing milkman. There's no telling what concept or anecdote might accidentally arouse a previously undiscovered kink in your libido. Far be it from me to delay the pleasure any longer. Dive in. Flip around. Thumb through. Open yourself up to whatever may come and let the universe have its way with you.

—JAMIE BUFALINO
DECEMBER 2007

In addition to being New York City's reigning sexpert since the 1998 launch of his "Get Naked" column in *Time Out New York*, Jamie Bufalino is currently a senior editor at *People* magazine.

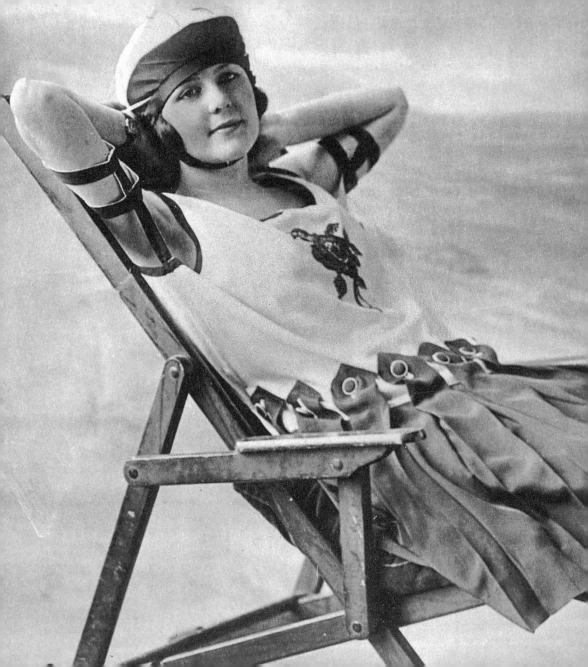

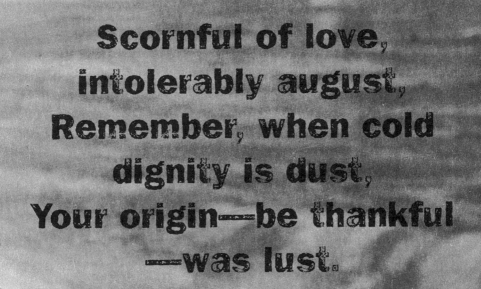

**Scornful of love,
intolerably august,
Remember, when cold
dignity is dust,
Your origin—be thankful
—was lust.**

—Palladas (4th c. Greek poet)

HELLO TWELVE

by Edward Kleban

VAL: Hello twelve.

RICHIE: Hello thirteen.

MAGGIE: Hello love.

AL: Changes, oh!

BEBE: Down below.

DIANA: Up above.

VAL: Time to doubt.

MIKE: To break out.

RICHIE: It's a mess.

MAGGIE: It's a mess.

PAUL & JUDY: Time to grow.

MAGGIE & AL: Time to go.

CONNIE, BOBBY & RICHIE: Adolesce.

ALL: Adolesce. Too young to take over, Too old to ignore.

AL: Gee, I'm almost ready.

ALL: But . . . what . . . for? There's a lot I am not certain of. Hello twelve, hello thirteen, hello love.

(Lights come up on group who are back on line)

CONNIE *(Stepping forward and singing)*: Four foot ten. Four foot ten. That's the story of my life. I remember when every body was my size. Boy, was that great. But then everybody started moving up and—there I was, stuck at . . . Four foot ten. Four foot ten. But I kept hoping and praying. I used to hang from a parallel bar by the hour, hoping I'd stretch just an inch more. 'Cause I was into dancing then, and I was good. And I wanted so much to grow up to be a prima ballerina. Then I went out for . . . CHEERLEADER! And they told me: "No dice, you'll get lost on the football field. The pom-poms are bigger than you." I spent my whole childhood waiting to grow . . .

(CONNIE goes into pantomime. The others have moved to dance formation. Each solo is picked up by spotlight)

VAL: Tits! When am I gonna grow tits?

PAUL: Secret, my whole life was a secret.

MIKE: One little fart! . . . And they called me Stinky for three years. Aahhh!

ALL *(except CONNIE)*: Goodbye twelve, goodbye thirteen, hello love . . .

BEBE: Robert Goulet, Robert Goulet, my God, Robert Goulet!

DON: Playing doctor with Evelyn.

RICHIE: I'll show you mine, you show me yours.

KRISTINE: Seeing Daddy . . . naked!

ALL: Time to grow, time to go . . .

SHEILA: Surprise! Mom and Dad were doing it.

BOBBY: I'm gonna be a movie star.

CONNIE *(Out of pantomime. The rest of the cast is now back on the line and lights come up)*: But you see, the only thing about me that grew was my desire. I was never gonna be Maria Tallchief. I was just . . . this peanut on pointe! That was my whole trip—my size. It still is. God, my last show I was thirty-two and I played a fourteen-year-old brat . . . And I shouldn't knock it 'cause I've always been able to work . . . From the time I was five in *King and I*, up 'til now I've never stopped 'cause whatever I am I am.

(Don enters upstage right, crosses down below line)

DON: The summer I turned fifteen, I lied about my age so I could join AGVA—you know . . . The night club union, 'cause I could make sixty dollars a week working these strip joints outside of Kansas City. I worked this one club for about eight weeks straight and I really became friendly with this stripper. Her name was Lola Latores and her dynamic, twin forty-fours. Well, she really took to me. I mean, we did share the *only* dressing room, and she did a lot of dressing . . . Anyway, she used to come and pick me up and drive me to work nights. Well, the neighbors would all be hanging outside of their windows, and she'd drive up in her pink Cadillac convertible and . . . smile. And I'd come tripping out of the house in my little tuxedo and my tap shoes in my hand and we'd drive off down the block with her long, flaming red hair just blowing in the wind.

(DON goes into pantomime and the other line people enter stage left. Each soloist is picked up in head spot as they sing their lines)

ALL: Goodbye twelve, goodbye thirteen, hello love.

MAGGIE: Why do I pay for all those lessons? Dance for Gran'ma! Dance for Gran'ma!

BEBE: My God, that Steve McQueen's real sexy, Bob Goulet out, Steve McQueen in!

CASSIE: You cannot go to the movies until you finish your homework.

AL: Wash the car.

MIKE: Stop pickin' your nose.

MAGGIE: Oh, darling, you're not old enough to wear a bra. You've got nothing to hold it up.

MARK: Locked in the bathroom with *Peyton Place*.

VAL: Tits! When am I gonna grow tits?

BOBBY: If Troy Donahue could be a movie star, then I could be a movie star.

DON *(Out of pantomime)*: Well, when the guys on the block saw Lola, they all wanted to know what the story was, and I told them about this big hot romance we were having, but actually she was going with this . . .

(DON steps upstage into darkness and joins group and Judy moves forward from upstage left)

JUDY: But my mother would embarrass me so when she'd come to pick me up at school with all those great, big, yellow rollers in her hair no matter how much I begged her and she'd say: "What are you, ashamed of your own mother?" But the thing that made my daddy laugh so much was when I used to jump and dance around the living room . . . *(Judy goes into pantomime)*

MAGGIE: Please take this message to Mother from me. Carry it with you across the blue sea. "Mother, oh, Mother, wherever I go your Maggie is missin' you so."

AL: Dad would take Mom to Roseland. She'd come home with her shoes in her hand.

DIANA: Mama fat, always in the kitchen cooking all the time.

SHEILA: Darling, I can tell you now, your father went through life with an open fly.

VAL: Tits! Where are my tits?

CASSIE: Listen to your mother. Those stage and movie people got there because they're special.

GREG: You take after your father's side of the family, the ugly side.

PAUL: Wait until your father gets home.

DON: Swear to God and hope to die . . .

JUDY *(Out of pantomime)*: And it was the first time I'd ever seen a dead body. But then when I was fifteen the most terrible thing happened. The Ted

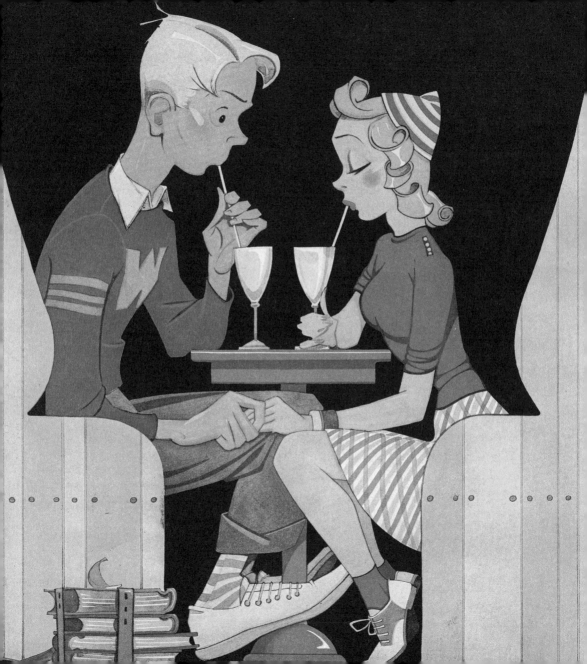

Mack Amateur Hour held auditions in St. Louie and I didn't hear about it 'til after they'd gone and I nearly killed myself. I tried to walk in front of a speeding streetcar and I remember noticing boys for the first time. Anyway, I remember practicing kissing with Leslie. She was my best girl friend. Did any of you ever practice kissing with another girl . . . So that when the time came you'd know how to? *(Listens, then speaks)* No? . . . Oh my god.

KRISTINE *(After a moment)*: Judy?

JUDY: Did you, girl?

KRISTINE: Yeah, but just a *couple* of times.

SHEILA: Oh, count me in.

JUDY: Thank God! *(Backing into line)* Anyway, I do remember . . .

GREG: *(Stepping forward)* The worst thing in school was every time the teacher called on me . . . I'd be hard, I'd be hard. Really, I'd have to lean up against the desk like this. And the teacher would say: "Stand up straight!" "I can't, I have a pain in my side." Or walking down the hall, you'd have to walk like this, with all your books stacked up in front of you.

MIKE: Yeah, I thought it was only me. I thought I was a sex maniac.

CONNIE & MAGGIE: You are!

BOBBY: I did too. I mean, it didn't go down for three years.

GREG: And the bus, the bus was the worst. I'd just look at a bus and . . . BINGO! And then there was the time I was making out in the back seat with Sally Ketchum . . . We were necking and I was feeling her boobs and after about an hour or so she said . . . "Ooohhhh! Don't you want to feel anything else?" And I suddenly thought to myself: "No, I don't."

ZACH: Did that come as a surprise to you?

GREG: I guess, yeah. It was probably the first time I realized I was homosexual and I got so depressed because I thought being gay meant being a bum all the rest of my life and I said: "Gee, I'll never get to wear nice clothes . . ." And I was really into clothes, I had this pair of powder blue and pink gabardine pants . . ." *(Greg goes into pantomime, the group breaks upstage from the line)*

AL: Early to bed, early to rise. Your broad goes out with other guys.

CASSIE: A diaphragm, a diaphragm. I thought a diaphragm was up here, where you breathe.

DON: I bought a car. I bought my first car.

MIKE: Padiddle.

MARK: Ev'ry girl I know has lockjaw of the legs.

CONNIE: You're not leaving this house 'til you're twenty-one.

KRISTINE: The ugliest boy asked me to the prom, I stayed home.

MAGGIE: Life is an ashtray.

VAL: Shit. Made it through high school without growing tits.

RICHIE: My trouble is wine, women and song. I can't get any of 'em.

MIKE: Your brother's going to medical school, and you're dropping out to be a chorus boy. Nothing!

BEBE: Steve McQueen out. Nureyev in!

DIANA: You gotta know somebody to be somebody.

MAGGIE: Grad—u—a—tion!

SHEILA: All you run around with are bums.

AL: I got Nancy's picture, Annabelle's locket, Cynthia's ring and Lucy's pants. Head-on collision! Eddie got killed . . .

RICHIE: Let's dance, let's dance.

PAUL: What am I gonna say when he calls on me?

JUDY: My only adolescence.

JUDY & KRISTINE: My only adolescence . . .

DIANE & BEBE: Where did it go? It was so . . .

VAL, DIANA AND BEBE: Where did it go? It was so . . .

GREG, BOBBY AND MIKE: Freshman, sophomore, junior, senior.

SHEILA, MAGGIE AND DON: Thirteen, fourteen, fifteen, sixteen.

MARK, CONNIE, CASSIE, RICHIE, MAGGIE, JUDY, PAUL, LARRY AND AL: Suddenly I'm seventeen and

ALL: Suddenly I'm seventeen and . . . suddenly I'm seventeen and . . . suddenly, there's a lot I am not certain of, goodbye twelve, goodbye thirteen, hello . . .

GIRLS: My braces gone.

BOYS: My pimples gone.

ALL: My childhood gone, goodbye. Goodbye twelve. Goodbye thirteen. Goodbye fourteen. Goodbye fifteen. Goodbye sixteen. Goodbye seventeen. Hello love. Go to it.

BOYS: And now life really begins.

GIRLS: Got to it.

ALL: Go to it.

(Music out; mirrors to black. The company is back on line)

—From the Broadway show *A Chorus Line*, 1975.

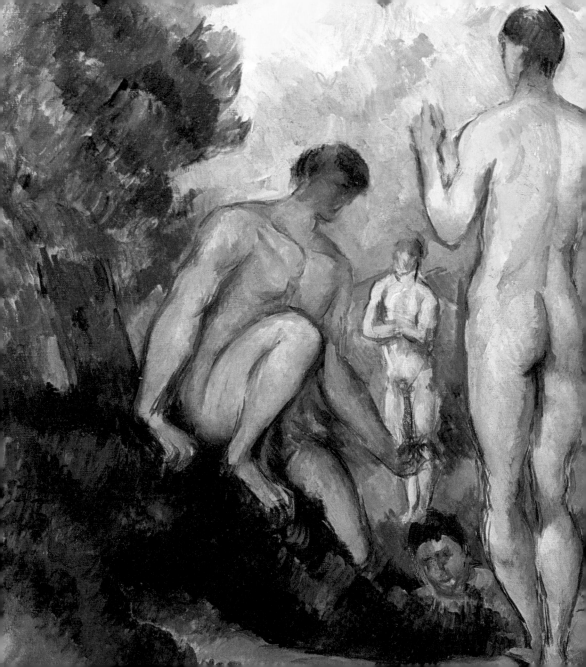

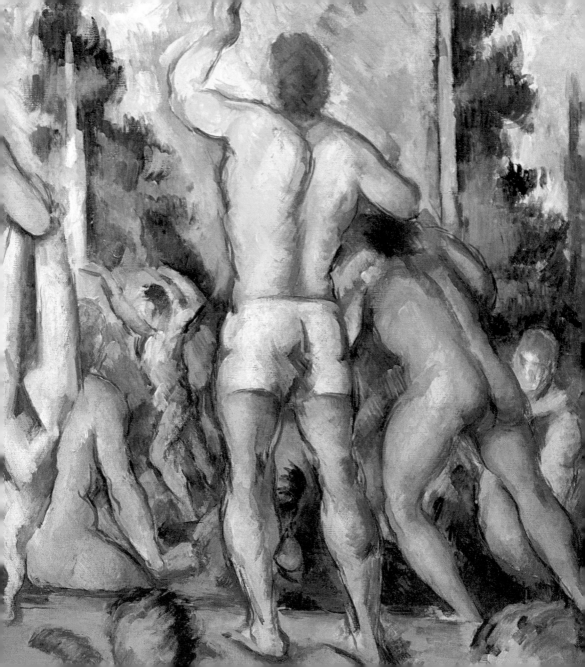

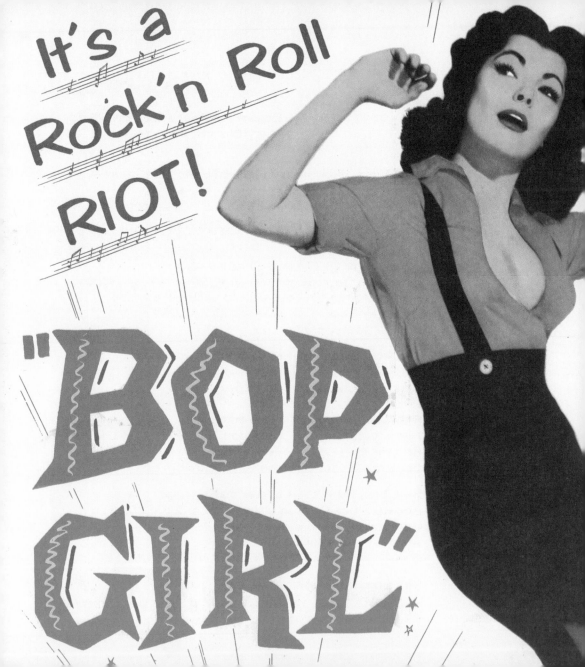

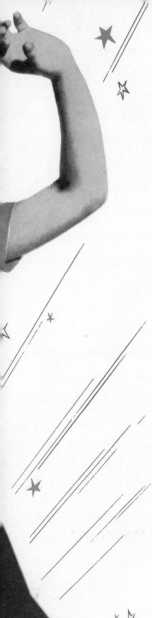

She Bop

By Cyndi Lauper, Stephen Broughton Lunt,
Gary Corbett, Rick Chertoff, 1984

Well I see them every night in tight blue jeans—
In the pages of a blue boy magazine
Hey I've been thinking of a new sensation
I'm picking up — good vibration —
Oop — she bop, she bop

Do I wanna go out with a lion's roar
Huh, yea, I wanna go south 'n get me some more
Hey, they say that a stitch in time saves nine
They say I better stop — or I'll go blind
Oop — she bop, she bop

She bop, he bop, a — we bop
I bop, you bop, a — they bop
Be bop, be bop, a — lu-bop,
I hope He will understand
She bop, he bop, a — we bop
I bop, you bop, a — they bop
Be bop, be bop, a — lu-she bop,
Oo — oo — she do, she bop, she bop

Hey, hey, they say I better get a chaperone
Because I can't stop messin' with the danger zone
Hey, I won't worry, and I won't fret
Ain't no law against it yet
Oop — she bop, she bop

She bop, he bop, a — we bop . . .

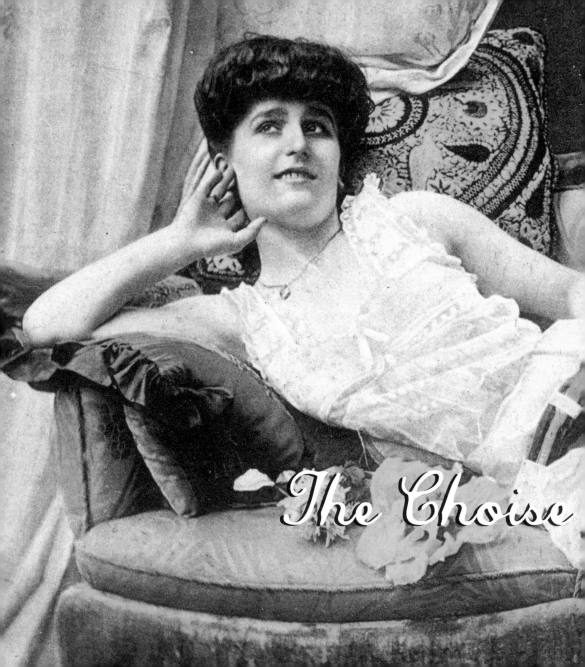

The Choise

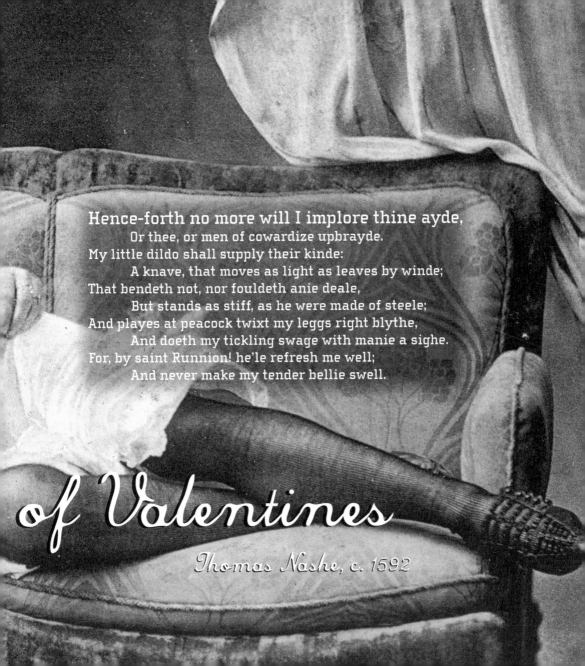

Hence-forth no more will I implore thine ayde,
　　Or thee, or men of cowardize upbrayde.
My little dildo shall supply their kinde:
　　A knave, that moves as light as leaves by winde;
That bendeth not, nor fouldeth anie deale,
　　But stands as stiff, as he were made of steele;
And playes at peacock twixt my leggs right blythe,
　　And doeth my tickling swage with manie a sighe.
For, by saint Runnion! he'le refresh me well;
　　And never make my tender bellie swell.

of Valentines

Thomas Nashe, c. 1592

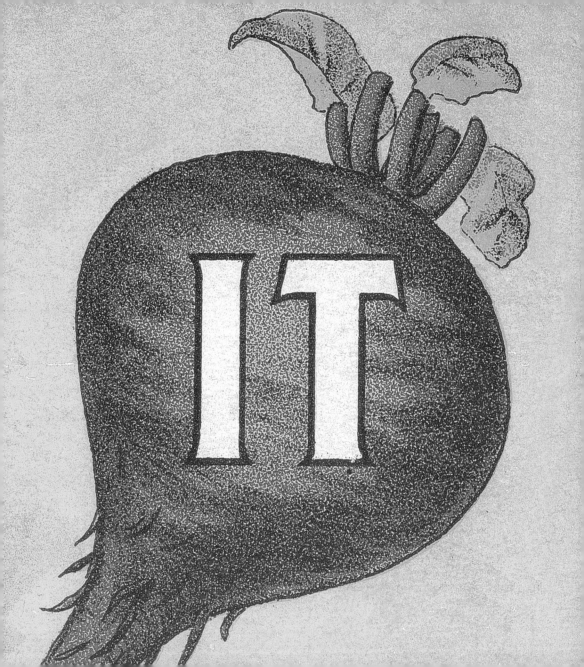

SOME THOUGHTS ON THE SCIENCE OF ONANISM

by Mark Twain

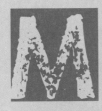

My gifted predecessor has warned you against the "social evil—adultery." In his able paper he exhausted that subject; he left absolutely nothing more to be said on it. But I will continue his good work in the cause of morality by cautioning you against that species of recreation called self-abuse to which I perceive you are much addicted. All great writers on health and morals, both ancient and modern, have struggled with this stately subject; this shows its dignity and importance. Some of these writers have taken one side, some the other.

Homer, in the second book of the Iliad says with fine enthusiasm, "Give me masturbation or give me death." Caesar, in his Commentaries, says, "To the lonely it is company; to the forsaken it is a friend; to the aged and to the impotent it is a benefactor. They that are penniless are yet rich, in that they still have this majestic diversion." In another place this experienced observer has said, "There are times when I prefer it to sodomy."

Robinson Crusoe says, "I cannot describe what I owe to this gentle art." Queen Elizabeth said, "It is the bulwark of virginity." Cetewayo, the Zulu hero, remarked, "A jerk in the hand is worth two in the bush." The immortal Franklin has said, "Masturbation is the best policy."

Michelangelo and all of the other old masters—"old masters," I will remark, is an abbreviation, a contraction—have used similar language. Michelangelo said to Pope Julius II, "Self-negation is noble, self-culture beneficent, self-possession is manly, but to the truly great and inspiring soul they are poor and tame compared with self-abuse." Mr. Brown, here, in one of his latest and most graceful poems, refers to it in an eloquent line which

29

is destined to live to the end of time—"None knows it but to love it; none name it but to praise."

Such are the utterances of the most illustrious of the masters of this renowned science, and apologists for it. The name of those who decry it and oppose it is legion; they have made strong arguments and uttered bitter speeches against it—but there is not room to repeat them here in much detail. Brigham Young, an expert of incontestable authority, said, "As compared with the other thing, it is the difference between the lightning bug and the lightning." Solomon said, "There is nothing to recommend it but its cheapness." Galen said, "It is shameful to degrade to such bestial uses that grand limb, that formidable member, which we votaries of Science dub the Major Maxillary—when they dub it at all—which is seldom, It would be better to amputate the os frontis than to put it to such use."

The great statistician Smith, in his report to Parliament, says, "In my opinion, more children have been wasted in this way than any other." It cannot be denied that the high antiquity of this art entitles it to our respect; but at the same time, I think its harmfulness demands our condemnation. Mr. Darwin was grieved to feel obliged to give up his theory that the monkey was the connecting link between man and the lower animals. I think he was too hasty. The monkey is the only animal, except man, that practices this science; hence, he is our brother; there is a bond of sympathy and relationship between us. Give this ingenuous animal an audience of the proper kind and he will straightway put aside his other affairs and take a whet; and you will see by his contortions and his ecstatic expression that he takes an intelligent and human interest in his performance.

The signs of excessive indulgence in this destructive pastime are easily detectable. They are these: a disposition to eat, to drink, to smoke, to meet together convivially, to laugh, to joke and tell indelicate stories—and mainly, a yearning to paint pictures. The results of the habit are: loss of memory, loss of virility, loss of cheerfulness and loss of progeny.

Of all the various kinds of sexual intercourse, this has the least to rec-

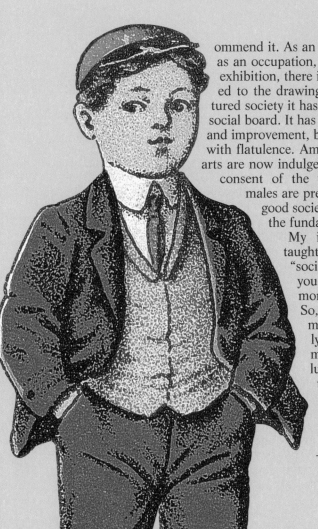

ommend it. As an amusement, it is too fleeting; as an occupation, it is too wearing; as a public exhibition, there is no money in it. It is unsuited to the drawing room, and in the most cultured society it has long been banished from the social board. It has at last, in our day of progress and improvement, been degraded to brotherhood with flatulence. Among the best bred, these two arts are now indulged in only private—though by consent of the whole company, when only males are present, it is still permissible, in good society, to remove the embargo on the fundamental sigh.

My illustrious predecessor has taught you that all forms of the "social evil" are bad. I would teach you that some of these forms are more to be avoided than others. So, in concluding, I say, "If you must gamble your lives sexually, don't play a lone hand too much." When you feel a revolutionary uprising in your system, get your Vendome Column down some other way—don't jerk it down.

—Mark Twain's speech to a gathering of the Stomach Club—a society of American writers and artists—in Paris, 1879.

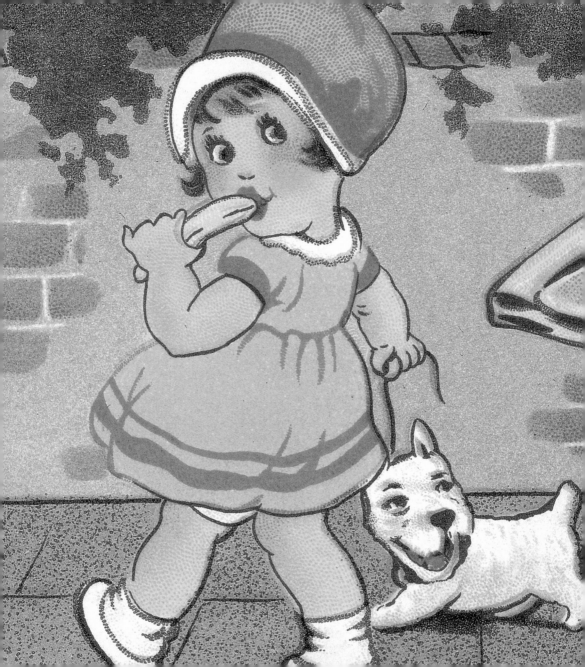

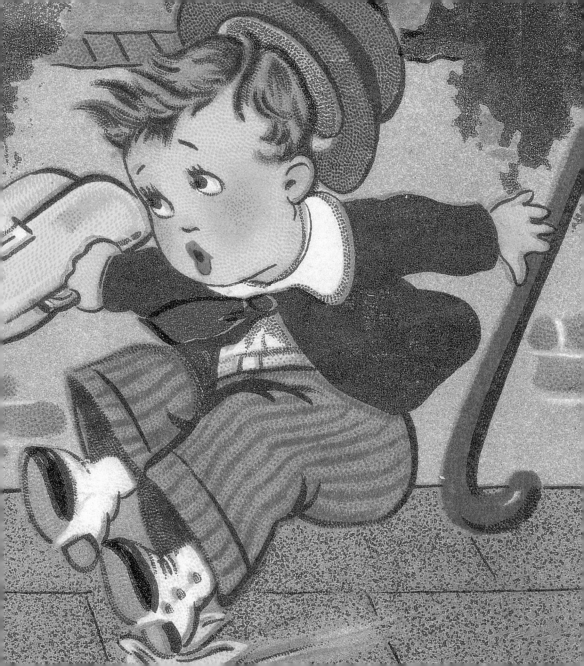

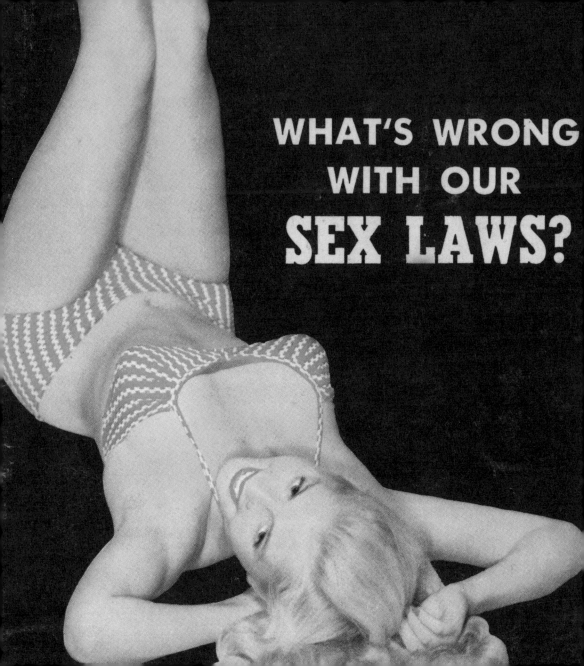

WHAT'S WRONG
WITH OUR
SEX LAWS?

Laws of Love

ARIZONA No more than two dildos are allowed per house

FLORIDA Only the missionary position is legal; sexual relations with a porcupine is illegal; men may not be seen publicly in any kind of strapless gown

GEORGIA One man may not be on another man's back in Atlanta

IDAHO If a police officer approaches a vehicle in Coeur d'Alene and suspects that the occupants are engaging in sex, he must either honk or flash his lights and wait for three minutes before approaching the car

ILLINOIS Attempting to have sex with one's dog is considered an offense

INDIANA It is illegal for a man to be sexually aroused in public

KENTUCKY One may not receive anal sex

MASSACHUSETTS A woman cannot be on top in sexual activities; taxi drivers are prohibited from making love in the front seat of their taxi during their shifts

MICHIGAN Couples in Detroit are banned from making love in an automobile un-less the act takes place while the vehicle is parked on the couple's own property

MISSISSIPPI Adultery or Fornication (living together while not married or having sex with someone that is not your spouse) results in a fine of $500 and/or 6 months in prison; unnatural intercourse, if both parties voluntarily participate, results in a maximum sentence of 10 years and $10,000; it is illegal for a male to be sexually aroused in public

NEBRASKA A man is not allowed to run around with a shaved chest in Omaha

NORTH CAROLINA While having sex, you must stay in the missionary position and have the shades pulled; all couples staying overnight in a hotel must have a room with double beds that are at least two feet apart; making love in the space between the beds is strictly forbidden; it is illegal to have sex in a churchyard

OKLAHOMA A man over 18 having sex with a female under 18 is statutory

Laws of Love

rape—provided she's a virgin; if she's not a virgin, then it is not a crime, but said person must be over 16; if both parties are under 18, then the law does not apply; it is illegal to have sex before you are married

OREGON Whispering dirty things in your lover's ear during sex is illegal

TENNESSEE Males may not be sexually aroused in public in Nashville

UTAH No one may have sex in the back of an ambulance if it is responding to an emergency call; in the town of Tremonton it is illegal to have sex in a moving ambulance; and if you are caught, the guy is let go and the woman is punished and her name appears in the newspaper

VIRGINIA It illegal to have sex with the lights on; one may not have sex in any position other than missionary; it is illegal for unmarried people to have sexual relations

WASHINGTON In the town of Auburn, men who deflower virgins, regardless of age or marital status, may face up to five years in jail

WEST VIRGINIA It is legal for a male to have sex with an animal unless it exceeds 40 lbs.

WISCONSIN A man having sex with a woman that is not his wife is considered rape; no male in Kenosha is allowed to be in a state of arousal in public

INTERNATIONAL

BOLIVIA It is illegal for a man to have sex with a woman and her daughter at the same time.

COLOMBIA In the town of Cali, a woman may only have sex with her husband, and the first time she does, her mother must be in the room to act as witness.

ENGLAND In Liverpool, topless saleswomen are legal—but only in tropical fish stores.

INDONESIA Decapitation is the penalty for masturbation.

LEBANON Men are legally allowed to have sex with female animals only. Sex with a male animal is punishable by death.

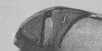

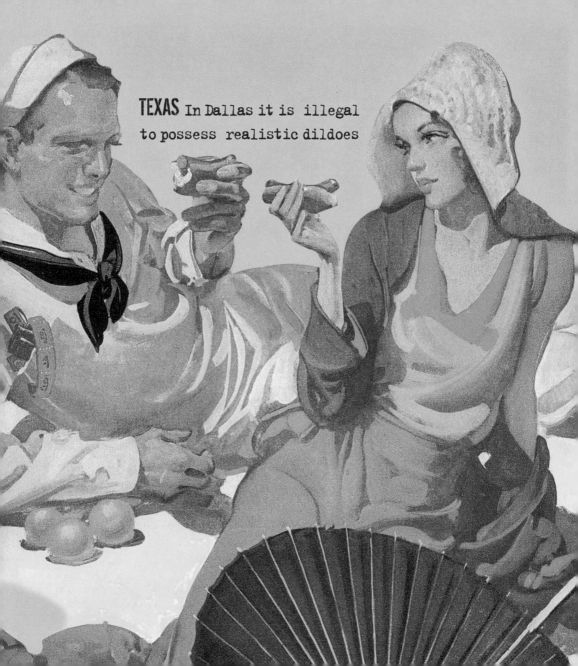

TEXAS In Dallas it is illegal to possess realistic dildoes

Ever since Eve plucked the fatal apple and Adam sunk his fangs in it, sex has been of uppermost interest to erring mortals. And one of the more interesting aspects of sex is the kiss.

How to do it?

Most primitive peoples perform the nose-kiss, not understanding how the mouth-kiss could possibly be of interest to anyone. . . . And yet these stone-age men and women do it with gusto.

Kissing can be fun, but it can also lead to a peck of trouble. Under certain circumstances, it is taboo, for instance in restaurants and parks, in some states, the theory being that kissing is a private affair.

There are other kiss taboos. When two women meet for lunch and kiss each other on the street, no one thinks twice about it. But except in France and a few other countries where these things are taken more lightly, if two gents meet and buss each other on the streetcorner, the law takes an unpleasant interest in the proceedings on the theory that there may be some kind of hanky panky going on.

Kissing can even be dangerous. Gangsters' molls among the Puerto Ricans of New York's Spanish Harlem have a clever little trick when they happen to find their guys unfaithful to them. When this happens, the girl takes a single-edge razor blade between her teeth, and then she receives her errant boy friend with a loving kiss that slices his tongue and lips like salami. Kisses can kill!

Art of Kissing

Lucrezia Borgia once murdered a series of lovers by holding a deadly poison in her mouth and then squirting it down their throats when they kissed. She was careful to wash out her mouth with an antidote afterwards.

But regardless of razor blades, poison, and the risk of catching colds, men and women seem unalterably addicted to the art of kissing. As the great Mohammedan prophet Abdul Fawzi ibn Sudani wisely wrote: "Mouloudji toh djarnah mouloudji!" Meaning: "The kiss is here to stay!"

—Excerpted from *He*, a magazine "For Guys With Guts," December 1954.

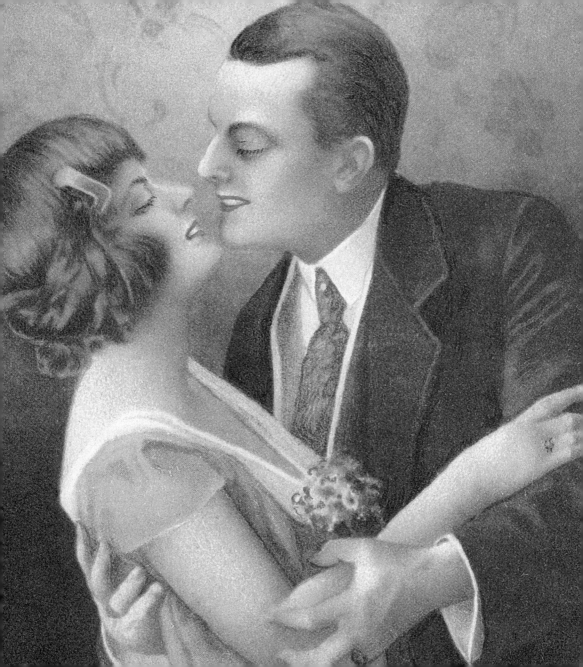

Hot Cross Buns?

According to historian and author Chris Roberts, seemingly innocent rhymes like the one about Jack and Jill or Goosey, Goosey Gander have more salacious origins. Jack's lost crown? His virginity. Goosey's lady's chamber? Turns out "geese" in 18th-century England was slang for prostitutes. As for Georgie Porgie, well, that was quite a sordid tale involving George Villiers (*aka* the Duke of Buckingham) and King James I who called him, "sweet child and wife."

With that in mind, what can be made of *My Son John*?

Diddle, diddle, dumpling, my son John,
Went to bed with his stockings on;
One shoe off, and one shoe on,
Diddle, diddle, dumpling, my son John!

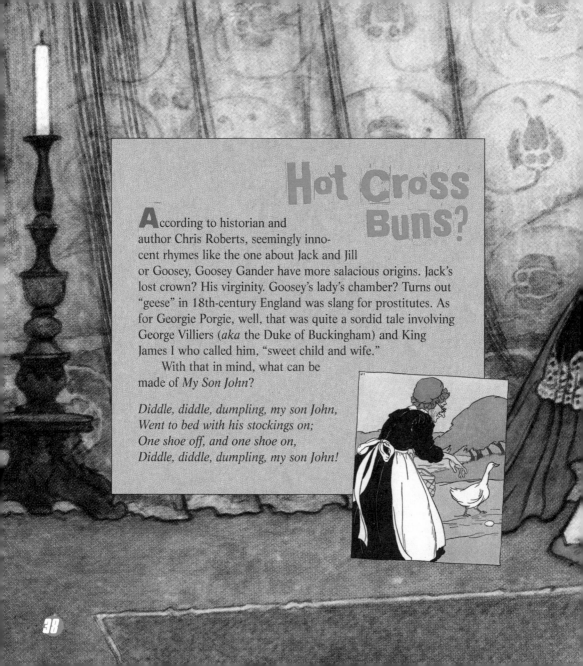

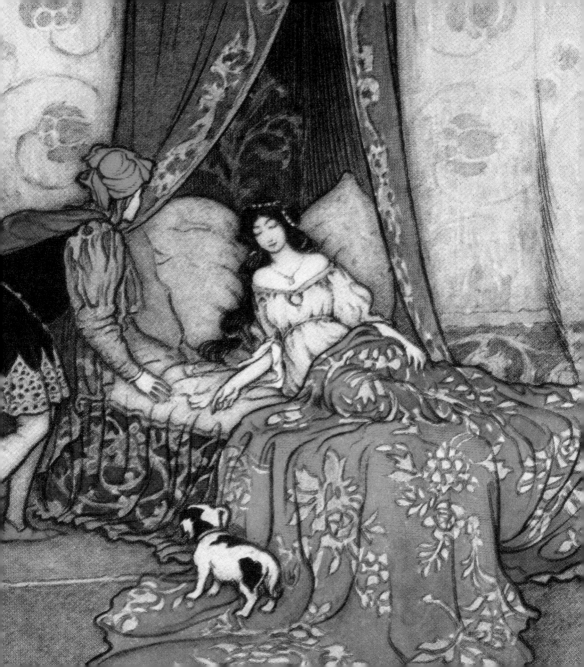

A is for Anatomical Correctness

(part one)

cock, prick, crank, rod, meat, drill, pud, tool, arrow, peter, wood or woody (erect), salami, creamsicle, pork sword, banana, baloney, shrimp tempura, cream filled sausage, oscar (My bologna has a first name . . .), egg roll, cod *gherkin* tube steak, lap taffy, meat and two veg, yogurt gun (or pump or slinger), love gun *goo gun* beef bayonet, beaver cleaver, single-barreled pump action protein rifle, heat-seeking moisture missile *tallywacker* pole, giggle stick, manrod, shaft, knob, happy pole, pipe, German helmet, Eiffel tower, John Thomas, willy, spanky, mickey, stiffy (erect), bologna pony, dong, mantower, twat jockey *pocket weasel* beaver buster, one-eyed wonder weasel, spunky monkey, trouser snake, zipper trout, jade phoenix *widow-consoler* wedding tackle (the whole package), cobblers (testicles), goolies (testicles), nuts (testicles), finger of love, grow-er (expands greatly; opposite of show-er), show-er (large when flaccid; opposite of grow-er) *third leg* womb broom, womb raider, cervix slammer, hector erector cervix inspector, tonsil tickler, gagger, jack the dripper, one-eyed milk man, pink-and-purple station wagon of desire, scepter *old boy* dork, tackle (genitals as a whole), manroot, boner (erect), choad, hard-on (erect), locker room terror (very large when soft), pecker *schlong* jack in the box (uncircumcised), spunk trunk, guided muscle, Johnson, sex driver, hose, bishop (refers to the glans of the penis, which is said to resemble a bishop's miter), skin flute, hooded knight . . .

J is for ___

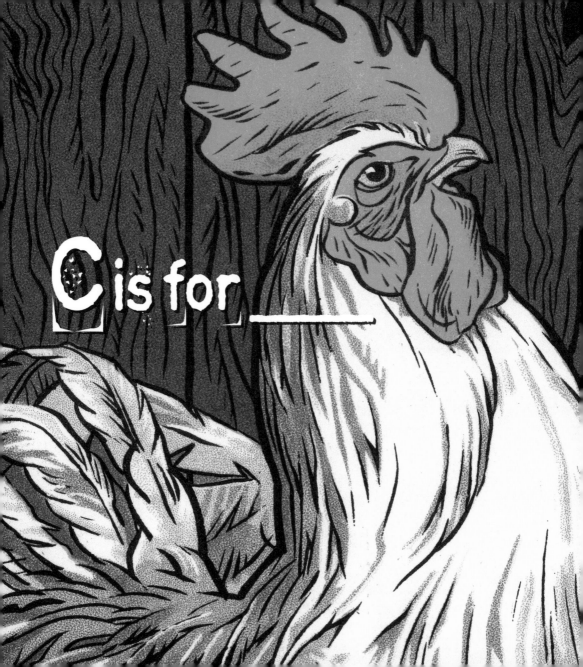

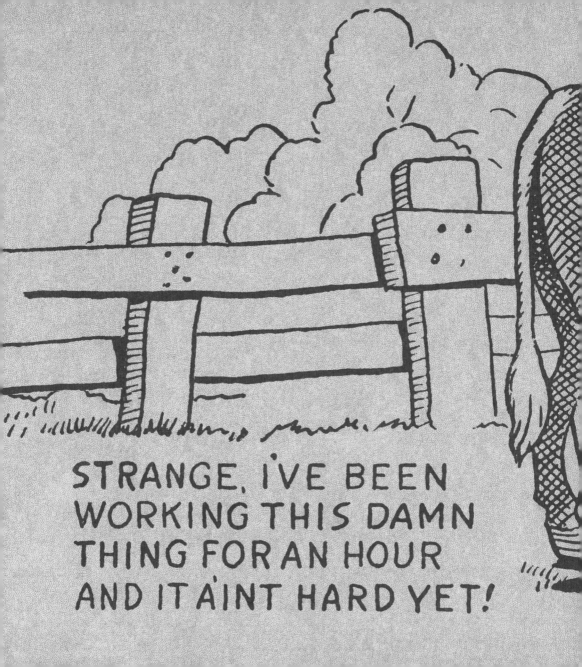

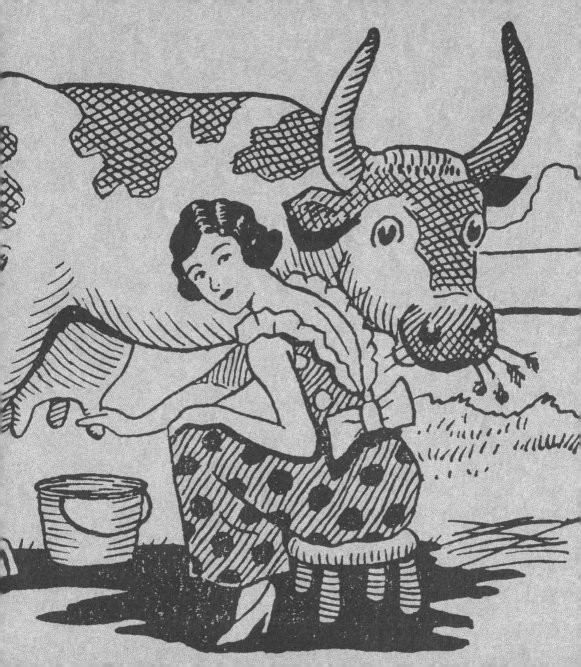

Bang! Up To Date

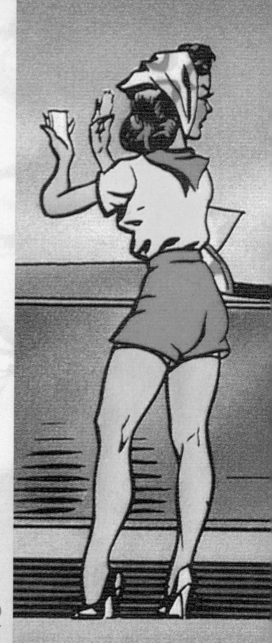

Harry tried to persuade Dolores to go for a drive with him in his 1951 Austin car.

"Sorry," she said. "It's too old-fashioned."

So Harry exchanged his car for a 1960 Ford.

Again Dolores demurred: "It's still too old-fashioned!"

In desperation, Harry lashed out and bought a 1969 Mercedes. Then Dolores was only too glad to go for a drive with him. When they reached a secluded spot, Dolores batted her sexy eyelashes and purred:

"Do you want to take my panties off, lover?"

"No, too old-fashioned," said Harry. "Spit out your gum!"

—From *There Was a Young Wench,* (1970) by Seymour Legge.

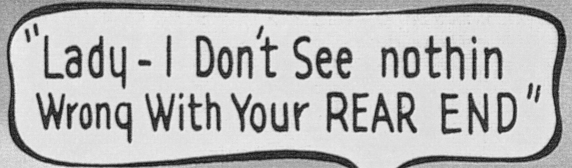
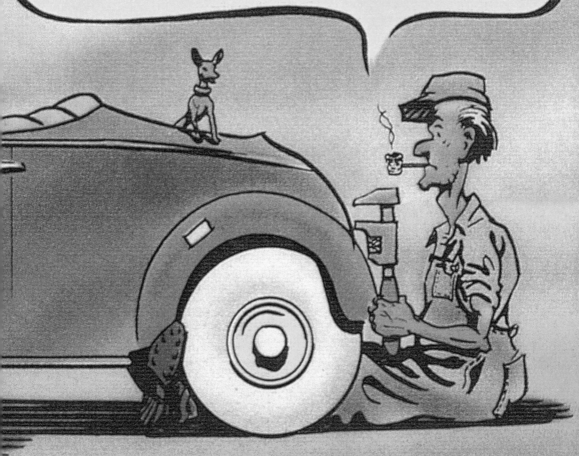

HOW TO MAKE LOVE

...if your arm is comfortably reposed across the girl's shoulders and "all's right with the world," then your next step is to flatter her in some way. All women like to be flattered. They like to be told they are beautiful even when the mirror throws the lie back into their ugly faces.

> Flatter her!
> Catullus once wrote:
> Kiss me softly and speak to me low;
> Trust me darling, the time is near,
> When we may live with never a fear
>   Kiss me dear!
> Kiss me softly, and speak to me low!

Tell her she is beautiful. Then take a deep sniff of the perfume in her hair and comment on it. Tell her that the odor is like "heady wine." Tell her that her hair smells like a garden of roses. Tell her anything, but be sure to tell her something complimentary. This done, it is only a natural thing for you to desire to sink your nose deeper into her hair so that you can get the full benefit of its bouquet.

—From the pamphlet "How To Make Love"
written by Hugh Morris in 1936.

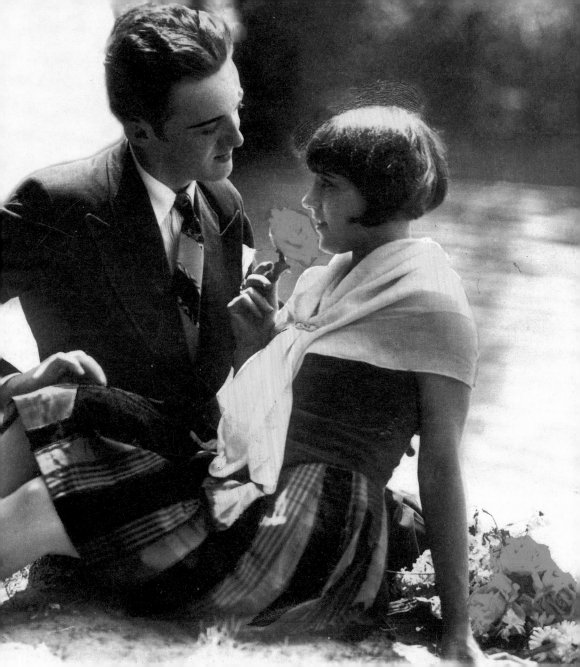

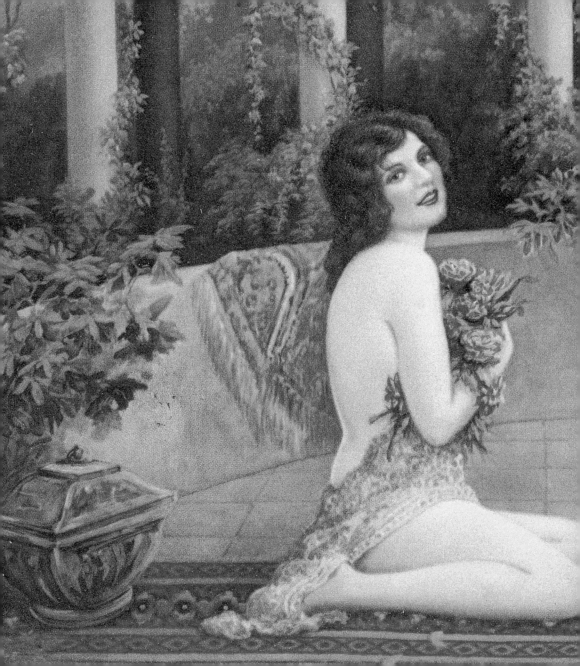

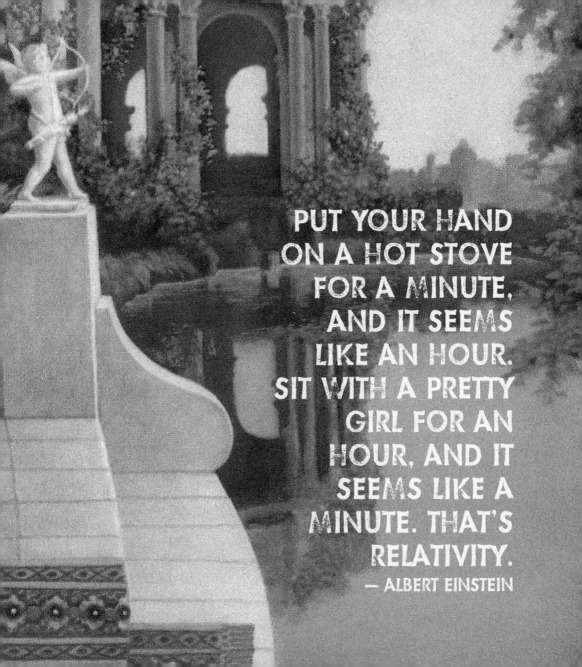

PUT YOUR HAND ON A HOT STOVE FOR A MINUTE, AND IT SEEMS LIKE AN HOUR. SIT WITH A PRETTY GIRL FOR AN HOUR, AND IT SEEMS LIKE A MINUTE. THAT'S RELATIVITY.
— ALBERT EINSTEIN

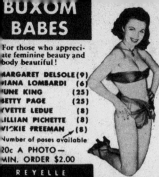
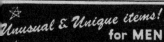
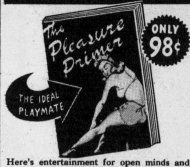
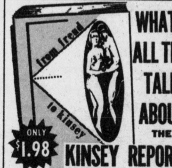

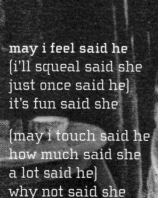

may i feel said he
(i'll squeal said she
just once said he)
it's fun said she

(may i touch said he
how much said she
a lot said he)
why not said she

(let's go said he
not too far said she
what's too far said he
where you are said she)

may i stay said he
(which way said she
like this said he
if you kiss said she

may i move said he
is it love said she)
if you're willing said he
(but you're killing said she

may i feel said he

e. e. cummings, 1935

but it's life said he
but your wife said she
now said he)
ow said she

(tiptop said he
don't stop said she
oh no said he)
go slow said she

(cccome? said he
ummm said she)
you're divine! said he
(you are Mine said she)

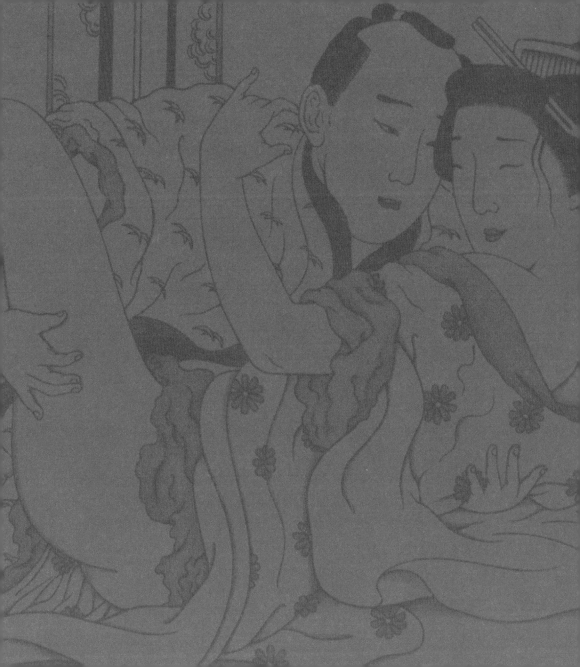

THE TALE OF GENJI

by Murasaki Shikibu

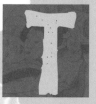

The governor of Kii was cordial enough with his invitation, but when he withdrew he mentioned certain misgivings to Genji's men. Ritual purification, he said, had required all the women to be away from his father's house, and unfortunately they were all crowded into his own, a cramped enough place at best. He feared that Genji would be inconvenienced.

"Nothing of the sort," said Genji, who had overheard. "It is good to have people around. There is nothing worse than a night away from home with no ladies about. Just let me have a little corner behind their curtains."

"If that is what you want," said his men, "then the governor's place should be perfect."

And so they sent runners ahead. Genji set off immediately, though in secret, thinking that no great ceremony was called for.

The east rooms of the main hall had been cleaned and made presentable. The waters were as they had been described, a most pleasing arrangement. The wind was cool. Insects were humming, one scarcely knew where, fireflies drew innumerable lines of light, and all in all the time and the place could not have been more to his liking. His men were already tippling, out where they could admire a brook flowing under a gallery. Having heard that his host's stepmother, who would be in residence, was a high-spirited lady, he listened for signs of her presence. There were signs of somebody's presence immediately to the west. He heard a swishing of silk and young voices that were not at all displeasing. Young ladies seemed to be giggling self-consciously and trying to contain themselves. The shutters were raised, it seemed, but upon a word from the governor they were lowered. There was a faint light over the sliding doors. Genji went for a look, but could find no opening large enough to see through. Listening for a time, he concluded that the women had gathered in the main room, next to his.

The whispered discussion seemed to be about Genji himself.

"He is dreadfully serious, they say, and has made a fine match for himself. And still so young. Don't you imagine he might be a little lonely? But they say he finds time for a quiet little adventure now and then."

Genji was startled. There was but one lady on his mind, day after day. So this was what the gossips were saying; and what if, in it all, there was evidence that rumors of his real love had spread abroad? But the talk seemed harmless enough, and after a time he wearied of it. Someone misquoted a poem he had sent to his cousin Asagao, attached to a morning glory. Their standards seemed not of the most rigorous. A misquoted poem for every occasion. He feared he might be disappointed when he saw the woman.

The governor had more lights set out at the eaves, and turned up those in the room. He had refreshments brought.

"And are the curtains all hung?" asked Genji. "You hardly qualify as a host if they are not."

"And what will you feast upon?" rejoined the governor, somewhat stiffly. "Nothing so very elaborate, I fear."

Genji found a cool place out near the veranda and lay down. His men were quiet. Several young boys were present, all very sprucely dressed, sons of the host and of his father, the governor of Iyo. There was one particularly attractive lad of perhaps twelve or thirteen. Asking who were the sons of whom, Genji learned that the boy was the younger brother of the host's stepmother, son of a guards officer no longer living. His father had had great hopes for the boy and had died while he was still very young. He had come to this house upon his sister's marriage to the governor of Iyo. He seemed to have some aptitude for the classics, said the host, and was of a quiet, pleasant disposition; but he was young and without backing, and his prospects at court were not good.

"A pity. The sister, then, is your stepmother?"

"Yes."

"A very young stepmother. My father had thought of inviting her to court.

He was asking just the other day what might have happened to her. Life," he added with a solemnity rather beyond his years, "is uncertain."

"It happened almost by accident. Yes, you are right: it is a very uncertain world, and it always has been, particularly for women. They are like bits of driftwood."

"Your father is no doubt very alert to her needs. Perhaps, indeed, one has trouble knowing who is the master?"

"He quite worships her. The rest of us are not entirely happy with the arrangements he had made."

"But you cannot expect him to let you young gallants have everything. He has a name in that regard himself, you know. And where might the lady be?"

"They have all been told to spend the night in the porter's lodge, but they don't seem in a hurry to go."

The wine was having its effect, and his men were falling asleep on the veranda.

Genji lay wide awake, not pleased at the prospect of sleeping alone. He sensed that there was someone in the room to the north. It would be the lady of whom they had spoken. Holding his breath, he went to the door and listened.

"Where are you?" The pleasantly husky voice was that of the boy who had caught his eye.

"Over here." It would be the sister. The two voices, very sleepy, resembled each other. "And where is our guest? I had thought he might be somewhere near, but he seems to have gone away."

"He's in the east room." The boy's voice was low. "I saw him. He is every bit as handsome as everyone says."

"If it were daylight I might have a look at him myself." The sister yawned, and seemed to draw the bedclothes over her face.

Genji was a little annoyed. She might have questioned her brother more energetically.

"I'll sleep out toward the veranda. But we should have more light." The

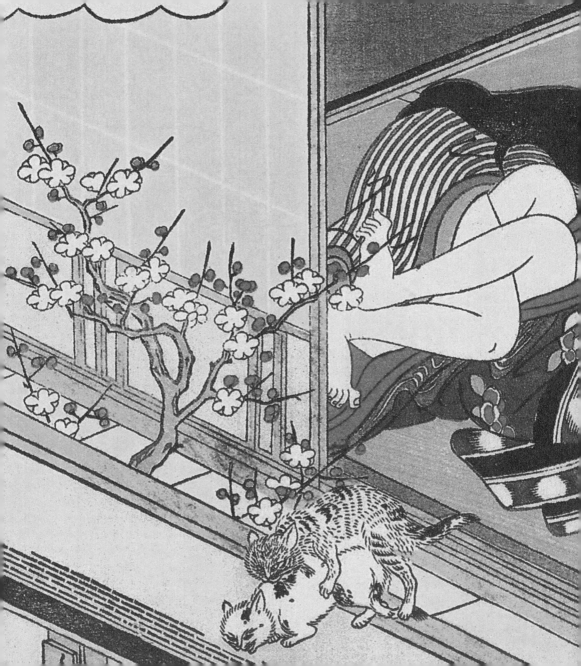

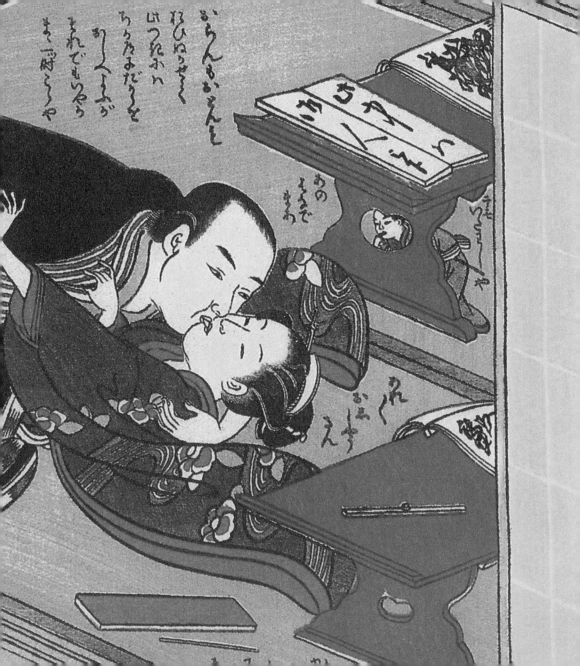

boy turned up the lamp. The lady apparently lay at a diagonal remove from Genji. "And where is Chujo? I don't like being left alone."

"She went to have a bath. She said she'd be right back." He spoke from out near the veranda.

All was quiet again. Genji slipped the latch open and tried the doors. They had not been bolted. A curtain had been set up just inside, and in the dim light he could make out Chinese chests and other furniture scattered in some disorder. He made his way through to her side. She lay by herself, a slight little figure. Though vaguely annoyed at being disturbed, she evidently took him for the woman Chujo until he pulled back the covers.

"I heard you summoning a captain," he said, "and I thought my prayers over the months had been answered."*

She gave a little gasp. It was muffled by the bedclothes and no one else heard.

"You are perfectly correct if you think me unable to control myself. But I wish you to know that I have been thinking of you for a very long time. And the fact that I have finally found my opportunity and am taking advantage of it should show that my feelings are by no means shallow."

His manner was so gently persuasive that devils and demons could not have gainsaid him. The lady would have liked to announce to the world that a strange man had invaded her boudoir.

"I think you have mistaken me for someone else," she said, outraged, though the remark was under her breath.

The little figure, pathetically fragile and as if on the point of expiring from the shock, seemed to him very beautiful.

"I am driven by thoughts so powerful that a mistake is completely out of the question. It is cruel of you to pretend otherwise. I promise you that I will do nothing unseemly. I must ask you to listen to a little of what is on my mind."

She was so small that he lifted her easily. As he passed thought the doors to his own room, he came upon the Chujo who had been summoned earlier. He called out in surprise. Surprised in turn, Chujo peered into the dark-

*chujo is the word for 'captain' in Japanese—Genji's rank.

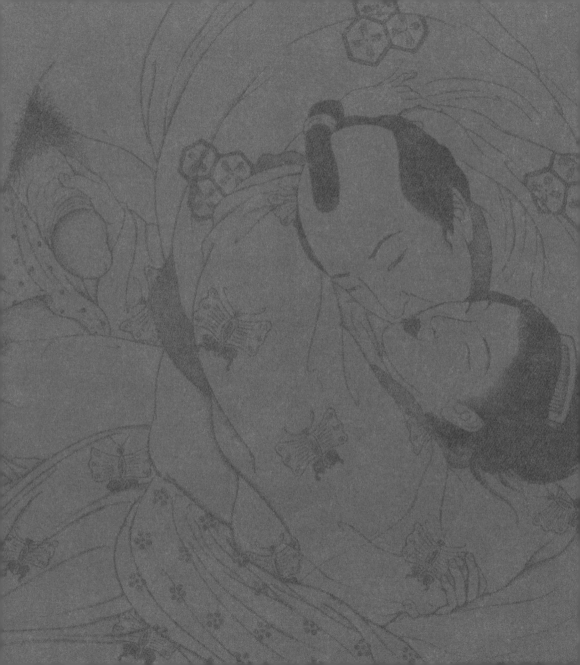

ness. The perfume that came from his robes like a cloud of smoke told her who he was. She stood in confusion, unable to speak. Had he been a more ordinary intruder she might have ripped her mistress away by main force. But she would not have wished to raise an alarm all through the house.

She followed after, but Genji was quite unmoved by her pleas.

"Come for her in the morning," he said, sliding the doors closed.

The lady was bathed in perspiration and quite beside herself at the thought of what Chujo, and the others too, would be thinking. Genji had to feel sorry for her. Yet the sweet words poured forth, the whole gamut of pretty devices for making a woman surrender.

She was not to be placated. "Can it be true? Can I be asked to believe that you are not making fun of me? Women of low estate should have husbands of low estate."

He was sorry for her and somewhat ashamed of himself, but his answer was careful and sober. "You take me for one of the young profligates you see around? I must protest. I am very young and know nothing of the estates which concern you so. You have heard of me, surely, and you must know that I do not go in for adventures. I must ask what unhappy entanglement imposes this upon me. You are making a fool of me, and nothing should surprise me, not even the tumultuous emotions that do in fact surprise me."

But now his very splendor made her resist. He might think her obstinate and insensitive, but her unfriendliness must make him dismiss her from further consideration. Naturally soft and pliant, she was suddenly firm. It was as with the young bamboo: she bent but was not to be broken. She was weeping. He had his hands full but would not for the world have missed the experience.

"Why must you so dislike me?" he asked with a sigh, unable to stop the weeping. "Don't you know that the unexpected encounters are the ones we were fated for? Really, my dear, you do seem to know altogether too little of the world."

"If I had met you before I came to this," she replied, and he had to admit the truth of it, "then I might have consoled myself with the thought—it might have been no more than self-deception, of course—that you would someday come to think fondly of me. But this is hopeless, worse than I can tell you. Well, it has happened. Say no to those who ask if you have seen me."

One may imagine that he found many kind promises with which to comfort her.

The first cock was crowing and Genji's men were awake.

"Did you sleep well? I certainly did."

"Let's get the carriage ready."

Some of the women were heard asking whether people who were avoiding taboos were expected to leave again in the middle of the night.

Genji was very unhappy. He feared he could not find an excuse for another meeting. He did not see how he could visit her, and he did not see how they could write. Chujo came out, also very unhappy. He let the lady go and then took her back again.

"How shall I write you? Your feelings and my own—they are not shallow, and we may expect deep memories. Has anything ever been so strange?" He was in tears, which made him yet handsomer. The cocks were now crowing insistently. He was feeling somewhat harried as he composed his farewell verse:

Why must they startle with their dawn alarums
When hours are yet required to thaw the ice?

The lady was ashamed of herself that she had caught the eye of a man so far above her. His kind words had little effect. She was thinking of her husband, whom for the most part she considered a clown and a dolt. She trembled to think that a dream might have told him of the night's happenings.

This was the verse with which she replied:

Day has broken without an end to my tears.
To my cries of sorrow are added the calls of the cocks. ■

—*The Tale of Genji* (c.1021) is often considered the first novel ever written.

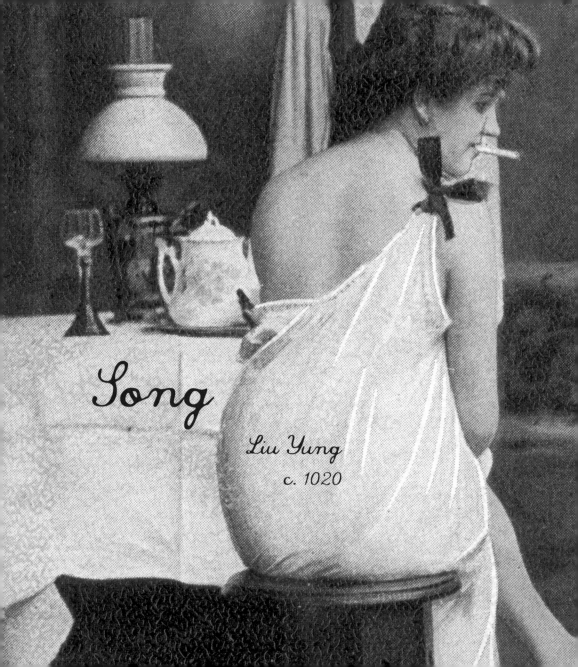

Song

Liu Yung
c. 1020

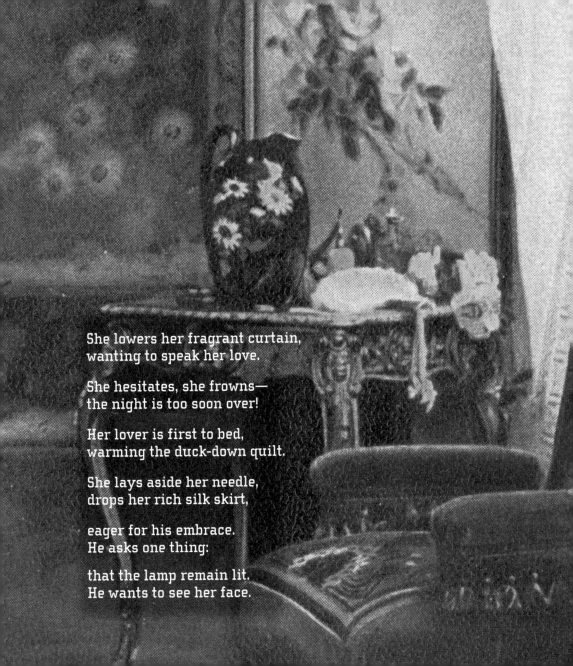

She lowers her fragrant curtain,
wanting to speak her love.

She hesitates, she frowns—
the night is too soon over!

Her lover is first to bed,
warming the duck-down quilt.

She lays aside her needle,
drops her rich silk skirt,

eager for his embrace.
He asks one thing:

that the lamp remain lit.
He wants to see her face.

The Language of Love

W hile "je t'aime" might get you some action in France, there is one custom that is advisable to follow wherever amour is found—using a condom. Lightweight, inexpensive and disposable, condoms may help prevent pregnancy and sexually transmitted disease. They come in a vast array of shapes, sizes, colors and even flavors, like chocolate, banana or mint. Here, in the language of love, are instructions for use. Remember: practice makes perfect.

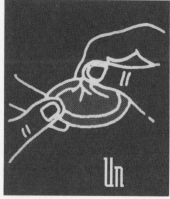

Un

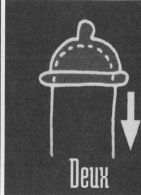

Deux

Conseils d'Utilisation

■ Utiliser un préservatif chaque fois que vous avez un rapport sexuel.

■ Le préservatif est à usage unique, ne pas réutiliser.

■ Ne pas utiliser le préservatif si la date de péremption inscrite sur la boîte est dépassée.

■ Mettre un préservatif avant tout contact entre le pénis et le corps de la partenaire afin d'aider à prévenir toute maladie sexuellement transmissible.

■ Ouvrir délicatement l'emballage individuel de façon à ne pas endommager le préservatif.

■ Prendre garde à ne pas déchirer le préservatif avec des ongles pointus ou

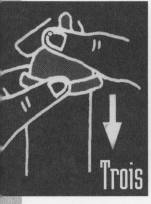

Trois

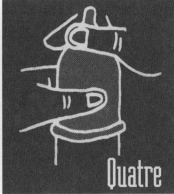

Quatre

lors du retrait afin qu'il ne reste pas dans le vagin.

■ N'enlever le préservatif qu'après le retrait total.

■ Après usage, le préservatif ne doit pas être jeté dans les toilettes. Mettre le préservatif usagé dans un papier et le jeter dans une poubelle.

coupants, des bagues et autres object.

■ Pincer avec les doigts le réservoir du préservatif afin d'en chasser l'air, le placer sur le pénis en érection.

■ Le préservatif doit être déroulé sur toute la longueur du pénis en érection. Attention à ne pas le dérouler à l'envers.

■ Cesser tout contact après l'éjaculation et avant la fin de l'érection.

■ Pour une plus grande sécurité, retenir le préservatif avec les doigts

■ Si vous désirez un lubrifiant supplémentaire, n'utiliser que des gels à base d'eau. Ne pas se servir de la salive, qui peut contenir d'autres microbes que le virus VIH. Ne pas utiliser de corps gras, de vaseline, d'huile; ils endommagenet le latex.

■ A ce sujet: nécessité de consulter son médecin ou son pharmacien en ce qui concerne des produits prescrits ou libres et destinés à être appliqués sur le pénis ou dans le vagin.

FROM *ARABIAN NIGHTS* (c. 900 AD)

■ Go to a hashish seller, buy 2 ounces of concentrated Roumi opium and equal parts of Chinese cubebs, cinnamon, cloves, cardamoms, ginger, white pepper, and mountain shiek (an aphrodisiac lizard). Pound them all together and boil in sweet olive oil. Next add three ounces of male frankincense in fragments and a cupful of coriander seed. Macerate and make into an electuary with Roumi bee-honey. Take a spoonful—washed down with sherbet made of rose conserve—after supping on mutton and house pigeon plentifully seasoned and hotly spiced.

A Hindu Technique for Dominating Women Sexually

■ Take pieces of arris root, mix it with mango oil and place the mixture in the trunk of a sisu tree. After six months prepare an ointment from the mixture and apply it to the lingam.

Vatodbhranta

■ For erotic stimulus mix together the following: vatodbhranta leaf, flowers thrown on a human corpse, the powder of peacock bones and the jiwanjiva bird; apply.

Camel Concoctions

■ Dip camel bone in the juice of the eclipta prostata plant, then burn it. Place the black pigment produced from the ashes into a box also made of camel bone. Apply the ash with antimony to the eyelashes using a camel bone pencil. This, it is said, will cause erotic subjugation.

■ Fat, melted down from the hump of the camel can be used as an aphrodesiac aid.

■ Mix honey with camel's milk and drink for successive days to produce marked potency.

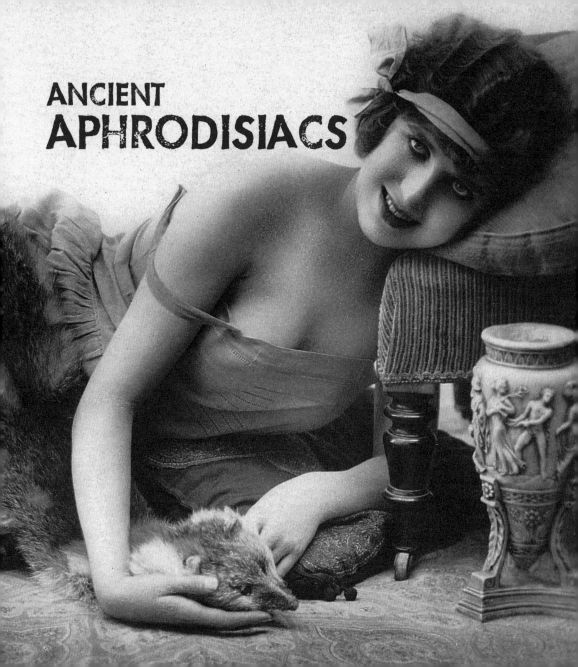

ANCIENT
APHRODISIACS

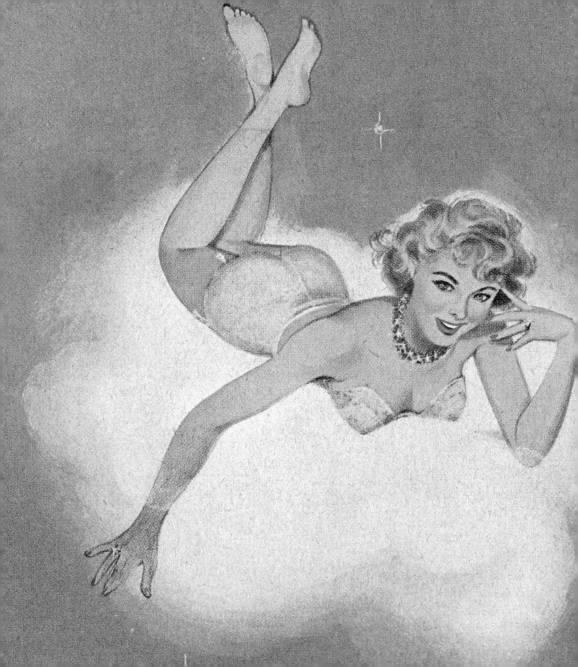

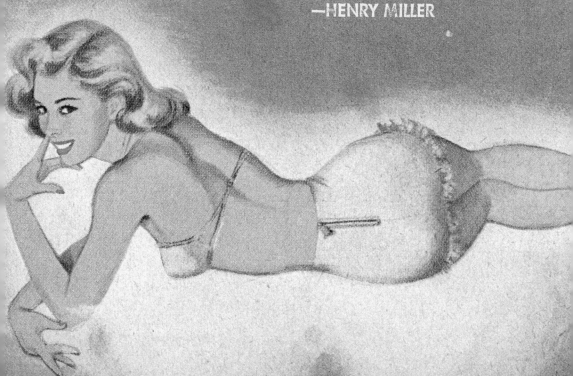

SEX IS ONE OF THE
NINE REASONS FOR
REINCARNATION,
THE OTHER EIGHT ARE
UNIMPORTANT.

—HENRY MILLER

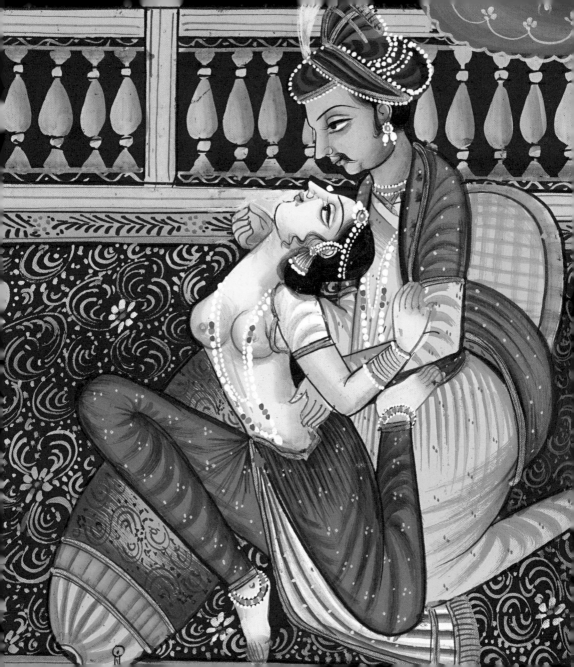

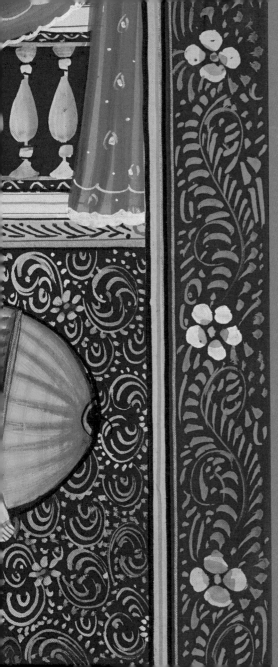

The Kama Sutra of Vatsyayana

Tradition holds that Vatsyayana was a celibate scholar who lived in Paliputra, India (modern day Bihar) sometime in the 4th century during the Gupta era—a cultural golden age that produced both the concept of zero and his most well-known work, the *Kama Sutra*.

Kama means desire, and *sutra*, discourse or technical text. His work is a compilation and simplification of earlier encyclopedic and inaccessible writings known collectively as *Kama Shastra* or "discipline of erotics." These works were attributed to Nandi, the sacred bull and doorkeeper of Shiva, who, upon hearing Shiva and his wife Pavarti making love, recorded their techniques in order to benefit mankind.

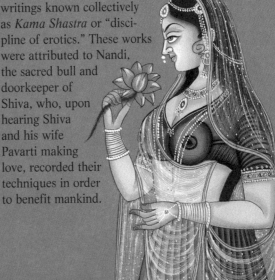

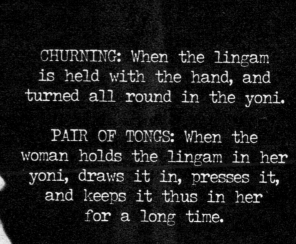

CHURNING: When the lingam is held with the hand, and turned all round in the yoni.

PAIR OF TONGS: When the woman holds the lingam in her yoni, draws it in, presses it, and keeps it thus in her for a long time.

TOP: When, while engaged in congress, she turns round like a wheel. This is learned by practice only.

Positions of the Kama Sutra

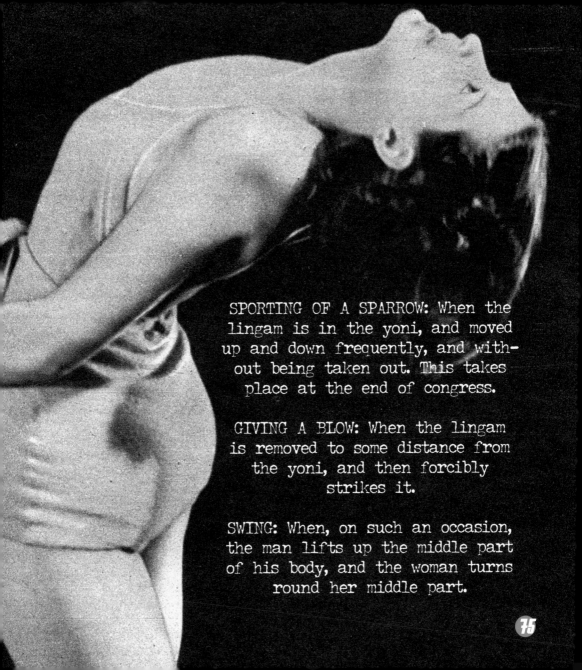

SPORTING OF A SPARROW: When the lingam is in the yoni, and moved up and down frequently, and without being taken out. This takes place at the end of congress.

GIVING A BLOW: When the lingam is removed to some distance from the yoni, and then forcibly strikes it.

SWING: When, on such an occasion, the man lifts up the middle part of his body, and the woman turns round her middle part.

A NIGHT IN A MOORISH HAREM

by Lord George Herbert

We were borne along at an unflagging gallop. Hasan held me in front of him like a baby in his arms, often kissing me, his kisses constantly growing more ardent; and then I felt his stiff shaft pressing against my person. He suggested that I ride astride for a while and rest myself by a change of position. I obeyed his suggestion, turning with my face towards his and putting my arms around his neck, while my thighs were spread wide open over his own. He let the bridle drop over the horse's neck, whose headlong pace subsided into a gentle canter which was like the rocking of a cradle.

Hasan put his arms around my loins and lifted me a little, and then I felt the crest of his naked shaft knocking for entrance between my naked thighs. I was willing to yield to Hasan anything he wished; but no sooner had the lips of my sheath been penetrated than I involuntarily clung more tightly around his neck and, sustaining myself in that way, prevented him from entering further. Hasan's organ seemed adapted to the place and excited a sensation of pleasure. I offered my mouth to Hasan and returned his passionate kisses with an ardor equally warm. A desire to secure more of the delightful intruder overcame my dread of the intrusion.

I loosened my hold on Hasan's neck; my weight drove his shaft so completely home, notwithstanding the tightness of the fit, that his crest rested on my womb. It felt so unexpectedly good as it went in that I gave a murmur of delight. The motion of the horse kept partially withdrawing and completely sending it in again at every canter. The first thrust, good as it was, was entirely eclipsed by each succeeding one. I could have murmured still louder with delight; but what would Hasan think of a girl so wanton?

But he was in no condition to think. He was fiercely squeezing and kissing me; while at every undulating movement of the cantering horse he seemed to penetrate me farther, and my womb was deeply stirred. The pleasure was too exquisite to be long endured. It culminated in a melting thrill, and my moisture mingled with the sperm that gushed from Hasan's crest. He reeled in the saddle, but recovered himself. The cantering motion drove his shaft less deeply in as it became more limber. It finally dropped out of me, a limp little thing drowned in the descending moisture.

"What a conquest for a slender girl to achieve over such a formidable object!" I thought. Exhausted, but triumphant, I laid my head on Hasan's shoulder. Twice more during the night he slackened the speed of his horse, and each time we completed an embrace equally satisfactory. ■

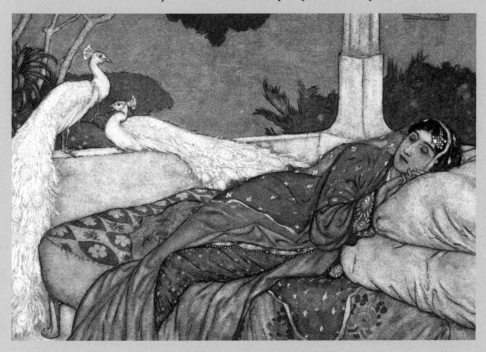

—Excerpted from the classic Victorian erotic novel first published c. 1904.

ALEXANDER THE GREAT (356 BC–323 BC): The bravest of warriors who always led his troops from the front, conquered not only Persia, but the Persian king's favorite eunuch as well. Historian Curtius describes the king's pet as, "Bagoas, a eunuch exceptional in beauty and in the very flower of boyhood." Alexander's best-known love, however, was his boyhood friend (and second in command) Hephaestion, whom he mourned for six months. Still, he had time to marry three times.

CALIGULA (12–41): Roman historian Suetonius wrote of Caligula: "He had not the slightest regard for chastity . . . was accused of homosexual relations, both active and passive, with Marcus Lepidus, Mnester the comedian, and various foreign hostages; moreover, a young man of a consular family, Valerius Catullus, revealed publicly that he had buggered the Emperor, and quite wore himself out in the process." He would also welcome Senators and their wives to an orgy, then ogle the wives "as a purchaser might assess the value of a slave," lead one to his bedchambers and return later to describe the tryst in detail.

Portraits in PLeasure

CASANOVA (1725–1798): Casanova bedded at least 122 women during his life, including a nun—in a three-way. Although acting as seducer was clearly his passion, church lawyer, violinist, chevalier, diplomat, and spy were some of his (non-sexual) positions. Duels, jails, escapes and banishments were everyday adventures. He earned fortunes and either lost (gambling) or spent (supporting twenty women in twenty households at once) it all. In the end he left countless debts and children scattered across the capitals of Europe—and had a great time doing it.

CATHERINE THE GREAT (1729–1796): Although she took many lovers during her reign (doling out great jobs and generous salaries), the story that she died while attempting sex with a horse (that fell on her) turns out to be idle gossip spread by those trying to put a powerful woman and very successful Empress in her place.

MARQUIS DE SADE (1740–1814): Jailed on and off throughout his life for abuses amounting to rape and torture—involving (amongst others) prostitutes of both sexes, chambermaids, his valet, and his virgin sister-in-law who had taken religious vows—the Marquis used his jail time to create most of his violently erotic writings. To this day his name is synonymous with that particular form of sexual gratification.

COLETTE (1873–1954): Leaving her first marriage, Colette set tongues wagging (and police raiding) when she planted a kiss square on the lips of her co-chorus girl/lover/niece of Napoleon III during a performance at the Moulin Rouge in 1907. A riot ensued. Her second marriage ended after a semi-public affair with her step-son, but her novels and short stories—often involving sex from a female perspective—became quite popular in the 1920s. Her most famous book, *Gigi*, was made into an MGM musical.

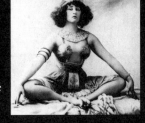

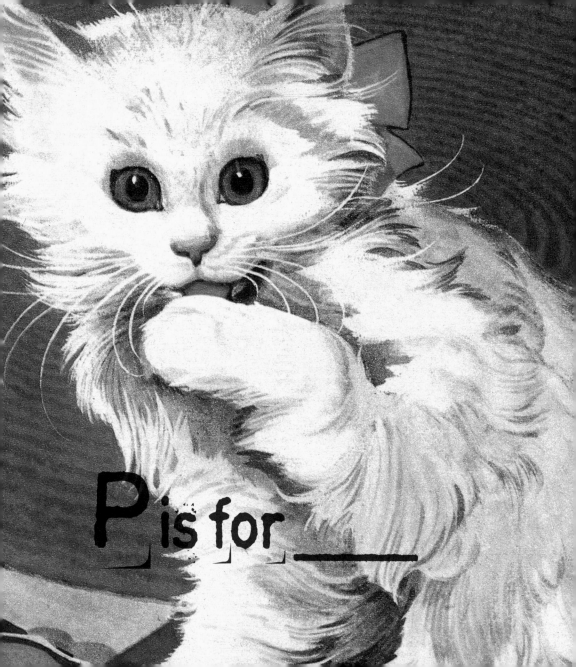

P is for _____

A is for Anatomical Correctness

(part two)

bearded clam, vertical smile, beaver, trim, tuna taco, cooch, cooter, punani, snatch, lovebox, box, poontang, pink cookie, love canal, flower, nana, pink taco, catcher's mitt, muff, roast beef curtains, whisker biscuit, carpet *love hole* deep socket, slice of heaven, the great divide, cherry, tongue depressor, honey pot, quim, meat massager, chacha, bush, fuzz box, fuzzy wuzzy, mound, peach, pink, love rug, snooch, pussy, kitty kat *poody tat* grassy knoll, cold cut combo, jewel box *rosebud* curly curtains, nether lips, altar of love, cupid's cupboard, love glove, spasm chasm, the condo downstate, breakfast of champions, wookie, fish mitten, pink circle, silk igloo, black oak, Republic of Labia, juice box *golden palace* skins, sausage wallet, holiest of holies, sugar hole, home plate, deer hoof, golden arches, cats paw, mule nose, yo yo smuggler, mumbler (Aussie), dinner roll *melvin* mumble pants (Sweden), ninja boot, marcia (Aussie), the big w, Chia hole, beetle hood, the Notorious V.A.G., furrogi (Poland) *little debbie* fortune nookie (China), pole magnet, pocket pie, clamarama, kitty cage, bubble gum by the bum, conch shell *crack of heaven* door of life, fruit cup, jelly roll, lobster pot, bunny tuft, knish, lotus, moneymaker, women's weapon, tackle box, bone hider, pizzo, toolshed, snake charmer *enchilada of love* furby, ham sandwich, Brazilian caterpillar, boy in the canoe, flesh tuxedo, mound of Venus, Venus butterfly, the helmet hide-a-way, furry 8 ball rack, crave cave, meat crease . . .

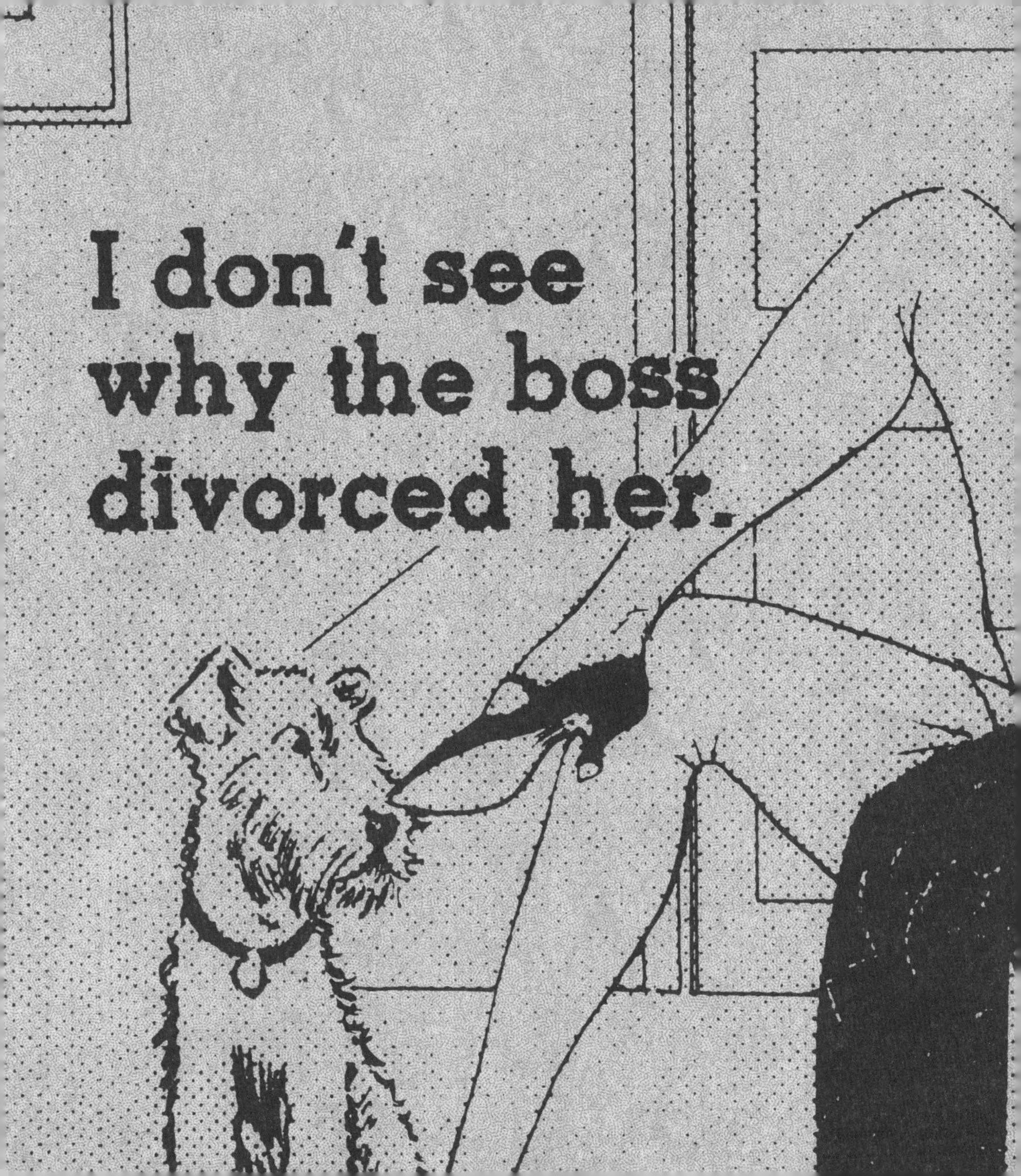
I don't see why the boss divorced her.

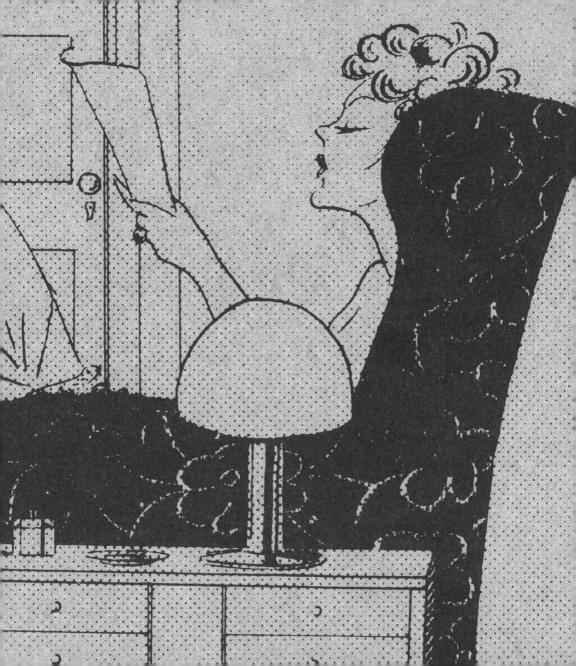

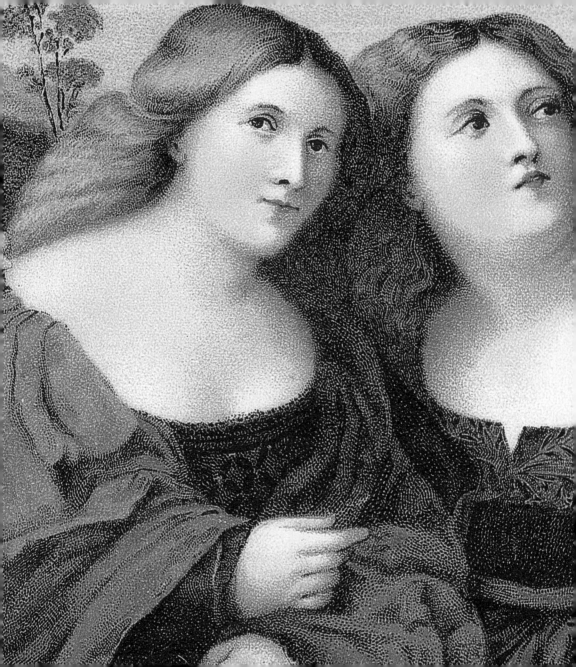

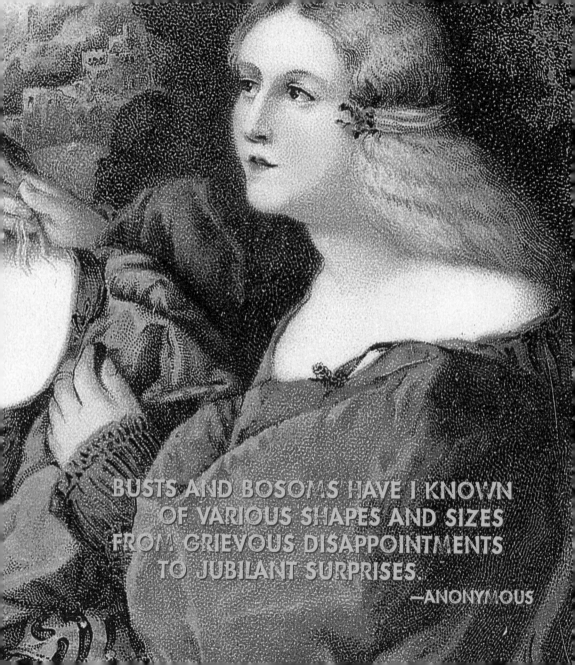

BUSTS AND BOSOMS HAVE I KNOWN
OF VARIOUS SHAPES AND SIZES
FROM GRIEVOUS DISAPPOINTMENTS
TO JUBILANT SURPRISES.

—ANONYMOUS

Bridget Asks:
Are You A Good Lover?

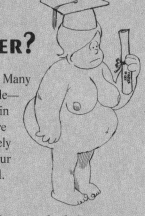

If you're a woman, perhaps the question sounds odd to you. Many women unconsciously associate the word *lover* with the male— but the truth is, women can and should take an active part in sexual relationships. How good a lover are you? Whether you're male or female, this simple, self-scoring quiz will tell you. Merely select the one answer to each question that comes closest to your experience and score yourself with the aid of the key at the end.

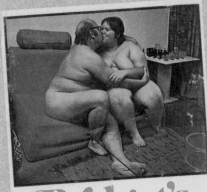

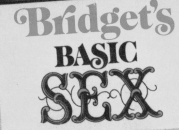

1. When you're having sexual relations,

❑ A. You figure it's up to your partner to divine what you like and act accordingly; and besides, you're not *sure* what you like;

❑ B. You know what you like, and you always let your partner know what pleases you most;

❑ C. What has liking it got to do with it?

2. Sex is best when

❑ A. You get it over quickly, in 30 seconds or less;

❑ B. It lasts as long as the mood dictates, and you're both in the mood;

❑ C. You thrash around for hours, until you both collapse in sweaty exhaustion.

— From *Bridget's Basic Sex*, 1977. Bridget in the Buff jigsaw, 1971.

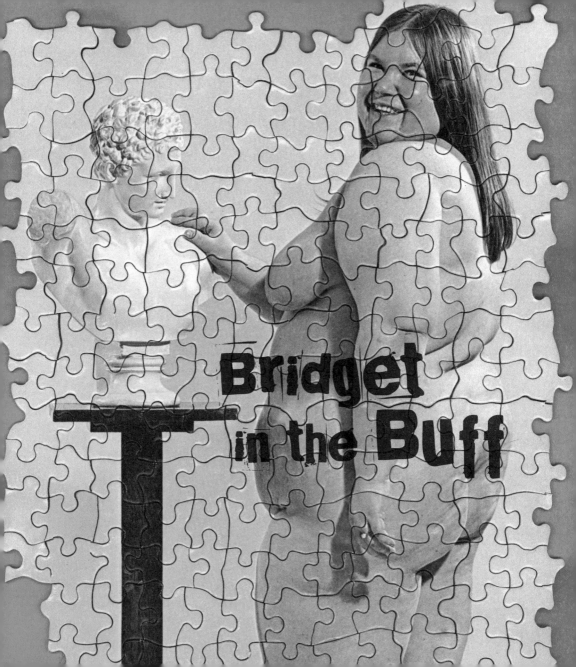

Bridget in the Buff

Bridget's Basic Sex

3. Sex with a stranger

    ❏ A. Is strangely exciting, particularly if you don't know your partner's name;

    ❏ B. Is O.K. sometimes, but you make it even better with your friends;

    ❏ C. Is the only time you can really let it all go.

4. Before sex, you . . .

    ❏ A. Always turn out the light and get under the covers;

    ❏ B. Enjoy looking and touching, and being looked at and touched;

    ❏ C. Like to get drunk, so you don't have to feel responsible for doing all those deliciously naughty things you like to do.

5. After sex you

    ❏ A. Always go to sleep;

    ❏ B. Like to relive the experience in your mind, savoring every ecstatic detail—while you rev up for another go;

    ❏ C. Usually wonder why people make such a big thing of it, when it's really such small potatoes.

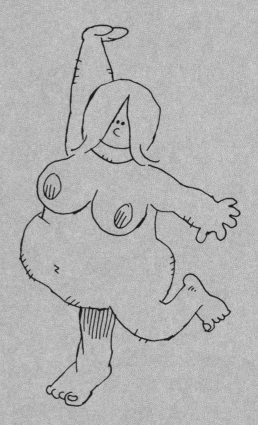

6. In the ideal sexual encounter,

    ❏ A. You are in control at all times;

    ❏ B. You are swept up in a huge tidal wave of emotion, deliciously out of control at the end;

    ❏ C. Your partner is in control at all times, and you like it that way.

7. Who initiates sexual relationships?

- ❏ A. You always do—you wouldn't feel comfortable otherwise;
- ❏ B. Sometimes you do, sometimes your partner does—and it's delightful either way;
- ❏ C. Your partner always gets the ball rolling, and that's the way it *should* be.

8. You achieve climax

- ❏ A. Mainly by thinking about it;
- ❏ B. Usually when your partner does;
- ❏ C. Tell me what it feels like, so I'll know if I've had one.

9. Oral sex

- ❏ A. Tastes terrible;
- ❏ B. Is a give-and-take proposition with you—and you like it both ways at once;
- ❏ C. Adds a little spice occasionally— but you wouldn't want it as a steady diet.

10. Your big worry over sex is

- ❏ A. If you're going to make it;
- ❏ B. That it feels so good you're afraid you might become addicted;
- ❏ C. Why worry?

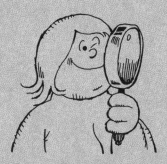

How to score yourself in quiz

Allowing one point for each of the ten questions, add up the number of times you selected answer b. Rate yourself as follows:

0–3 points It's a good thing you're reading this book—you need it.

4–6 points This is an average score, for someone who is scoring occasionally, but not very well. Too many nasty inhibitions. What can you do about it? Not a hell of a lot. But at least you found out in time.

7–9 points You've got a pretty good thing going—it's a cinch you're not getting much sleep.

10 points Congratulations—you're totally freaked out on sex. You'd better put this book down right now—before you really get in trouble.

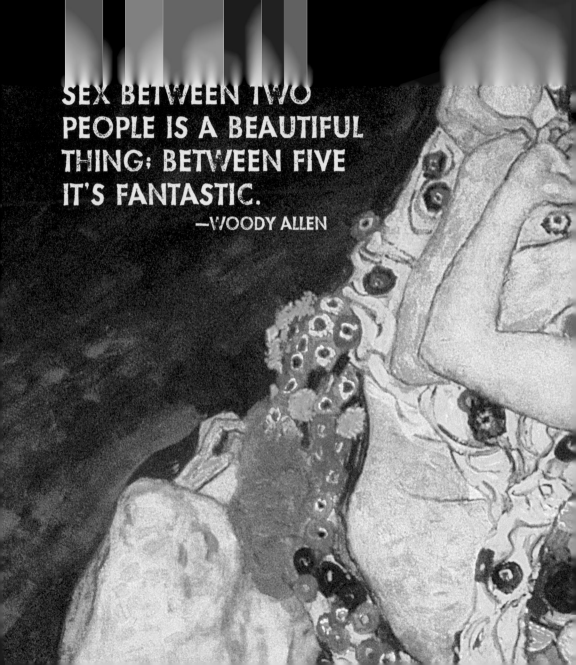

SEX BETWEEN TWO
PEOPLE IS A BEAUTIFUL
THING; BETWEEN FIVE
IT'S FANTASTIC.

—WOODY ALLEN

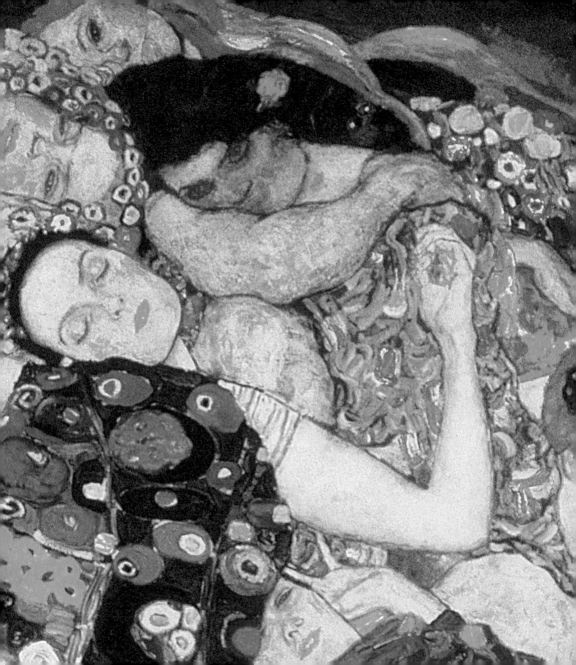

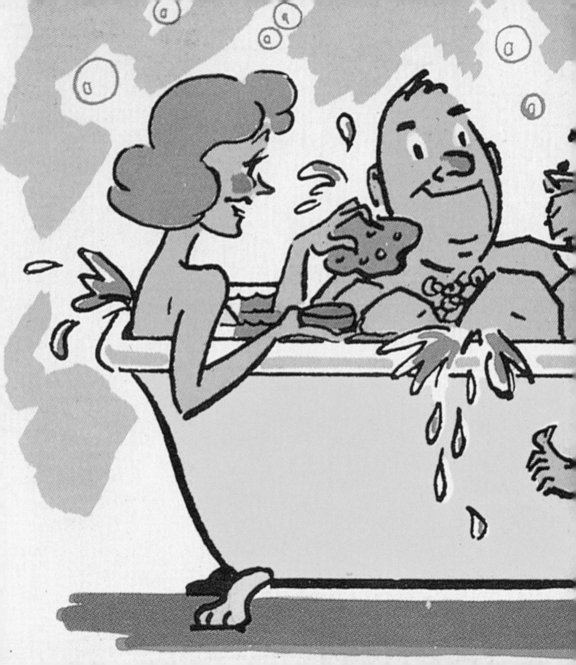

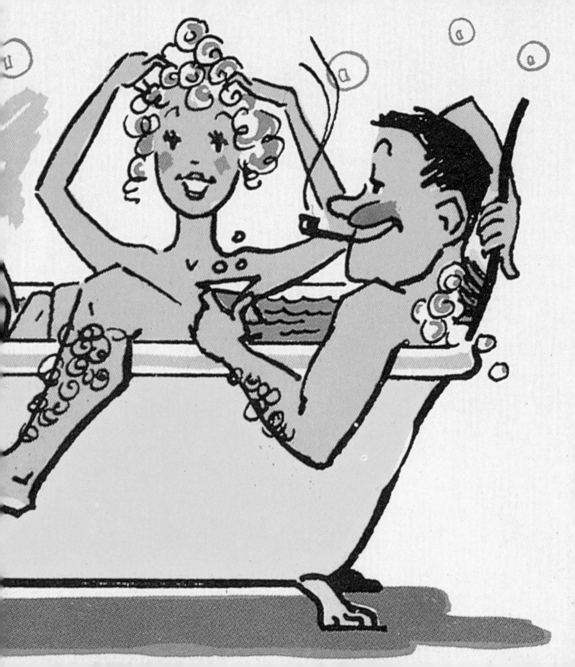

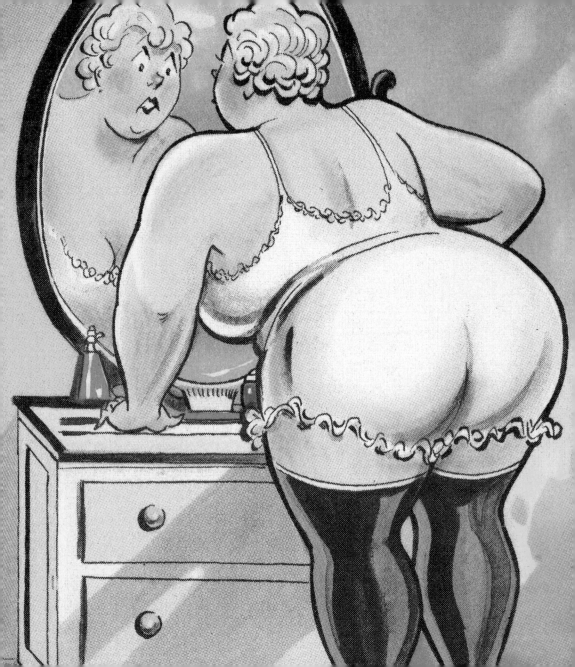

There once was a woman from Crewe
Who said as the Bishop withdrew
The Vicar is slicker
and quicker and thicker
and twelve inches longer than you.

There once was a deductive Brazilian
Who tinted her breasts bright vermilion.
Admiring her work
She said with a smirk:
"Caramba! They're two in a million!"

There once was a man from Racine
Who invented a loving machine
Both concave and convex
It could serve either sex
Entertaining itself in between.

There once was a queer from Rangoon
who invited a lesbian up to his room
they did argue and fight
all thru the night
as to who would do what to whom

There once was a plumber from Leigh
Who was plumbing a girl by the sea
Said the girl "Somebody's coming."
Said the plumber still plumbing
"If anyone's coming it's me!"

There once was a . . .

There once was a young maiden named Claire
Who was attacked by a bear.
While chased in the field
She tripped and revealed
Some meat to the bear that was rare.

There once was an lady from Brussels.
Accused of wearing two bustles
She said, "It's not true,
It's a thing I don't do,
You are simply observing my muscles."

There once was a girl named Ginter,
Who married a man in the winter;
The man's name was Wood,
And now, as they should,
They have a cute little splinter.

There once was a man from Nantucket,
Whose dick was so long he could suck it.
He walked down the street,
Swinging his meat.
While he carried his balls in a bucket.

'Twas the gath'ring o' the clans,
And all the Scots were there,
A-skirlin' on their bagpipes,
And strokin' pussy hair.

Singing, "Who hae ye, lassie,
Who hae ye noo?
The ane that hae ye last time
He canna hae ye noo."

Maggie McGuire, she was there
A-showin' the boys some tricks,
And ye canna hear the bagpipes
For the swishin' o' the pricks.

Sandy MacPherson, he was there
And on the floor he sat,
Amusin' himself by abusin' himself
And catchin' it in his hat.

The factor's wife, she was there,
Ass against the wall,
Shoutin' to the laddie boys,
"Come ye one an' all."

The mayor's daughter, she was there,
And kept the crowd in fits
By jumpin' off the mantel piece
And landin' on her tits.

The village idiot, he was there;
He was a perfect fool.
He sat beneath the oak tree
And whittled off his tool.

Johnny McGregor, he was there,
A lad so brave and bold.
He pulled the foreskin over the end
And whistled through the hole.

Down in the square,
The village dunce he stands,
Amusin' himself by abusin' himself
And usin' both his hands.

The elders of the church,
They were too old to firk,
So they sat around the table
And had a circle jerk.

The bride was in the corner
Explainin' to the groom
The vagina, not the rectum,
Is the entrance to the womb.

The queen was in the kitchen,
Eatin' bread and honey.
The king was in the kitchen maid
And she was in the money.

And when the ball was over,
The opinion was expressed:
Although they liked the music,
The fuckin' was the best.

The Ball

—Written in the 1880s to celebrate an actual "social event."

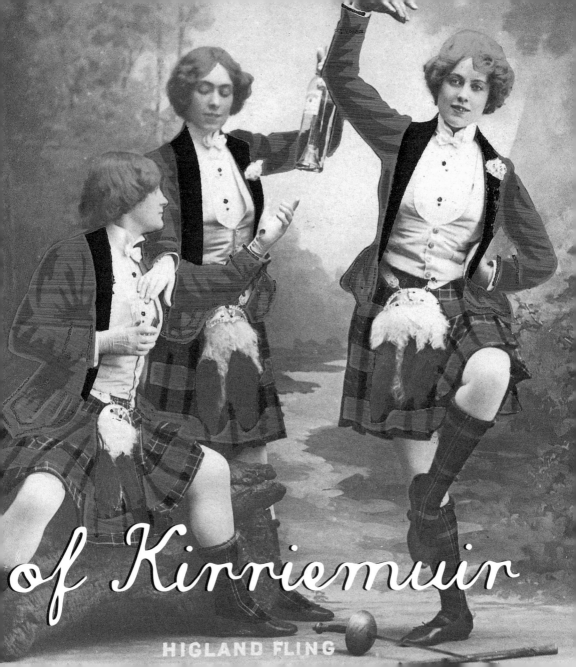

of Kirriemuir

HIGLAND FLING

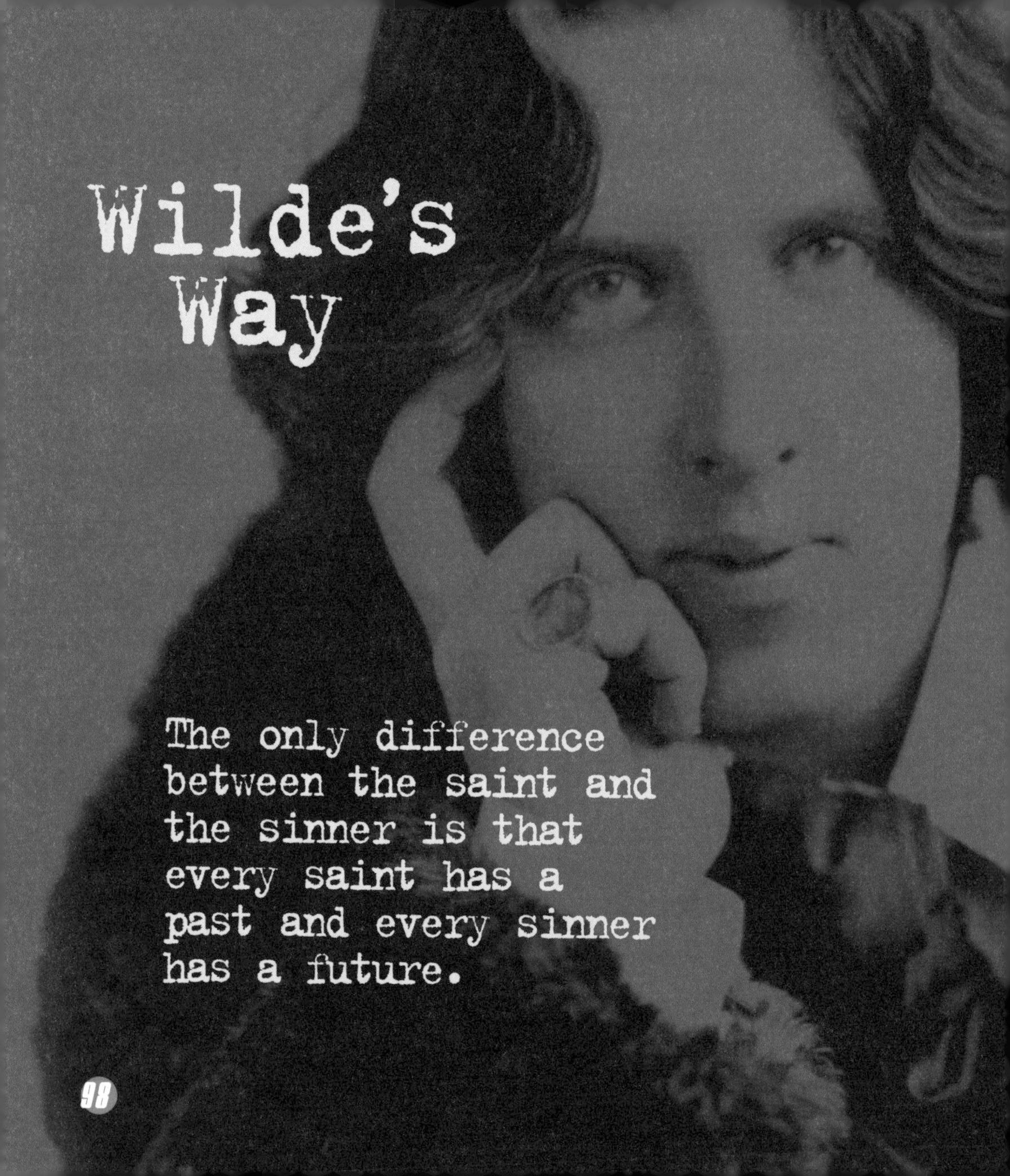

Wilde's Way

The only difference
between the saint and
the sinner is that
every saint has a
past and every sinner
has a future.

I do not play cricket because it requires me to assume such indecent postures.

I like men who have a future and women who have a past.

Women's styles may change but their designs remain the same.

The reason we are so pleased to find other people's secrets is that it distracts public attention from our own.

Don't be misled into the paths of virtue.

Men always want to be a woman's first love; women have a more subtle instinct: what they like is to be a man's last romance.

In married life, three is company and two none.

It was Oscar Wilde's provocative wit that got him into hot water and led to a conviction for gross indecency in 1895. After serving two years for, "the love that dares not speak its name," he fled to Paris. Buried in famed Père Lachaise Cemetery, the clearly-male angel on his tomb had his anatomically correct member broken off and used by a succession of guards as a paperweight.

ANGELA OF FOLIGNO (1248–1309) Until her conversion in 1285, Angela led a full, if lurid, life. Married with children she was also wild, adulterous and sacrilegious. While neglecting her duties as mother and wife, she made a transgression so grave that she couldn't even tell her confessor. The death of her entire family in one year and a vision of St. Francis of Assisi changed her. She confessed all to a Franciscan friar and later founded a community of sisters.

MARGARET OF CORTONA (1247–1297) Margaret had a mean step-mother and ran off with a dashing cavalier with whom she begat a son. After the cavalier was murdered, Margaret was tempted to trade upon her considerable beauty, but instead moved in with a group of Franciscan Friars. Unfortunately that did not prevent her from partaking in multiple sins of the flesh. To atone she became a vegetarian, started conversing with God and eventually established a congregation of Tertiary Sisters known as le poverelle.

MARY OF EDESSA (d. c.365) After 20 years as an anchoress, Mary—in a moment of weakness—was seduced by a renegade monk who had turned from his vows. In shame she moved far away and gave herself over to a wild, dissolute, and sexually active life. One day her uncle, the hermit Saint Abraham, decided to go forth (cleverly disguised as a soldier whom he knew she would pick up) and save her. Sure enough she took him home and there, over supper, he convinced her of the error of her ways. She converted, returned to the life of an anchoress and spent the rest of her days in prayer.

MARY OF EGYPT (344–421) Spoiled little rich girl, Mary ran away to Alexandria at the age of 12 to work as a singer, dancer and prostitute (although her biography states that she often refused the money offered for her services). "Insatiable desire and irrepressible passion" eventually drove her to Jerusalem where she hoped to supplement the meager income she earned spinning flax by selling her body. One day upon entering the Church of the Holy Sepulchre she was halted in her tracks by an unseen force. A glimpse of the Virgin Mary followed by a disembodied voice set her on the path to repentance and she spent the rest of her life as a hermit in the Syrian desert.

ST. PELAGIA (d. 284) Pelagia was a celebrated, beautiful and much bejeweled (but loose and wayward) actress and courtesan of Antioch, who at the height of her success—inspired by the preachings of St. Nonnus—gave up all comfort and luxury to live as a hermit—disguised as a man—in a cave on the Mount of Olives.

Sins
of the
Saints

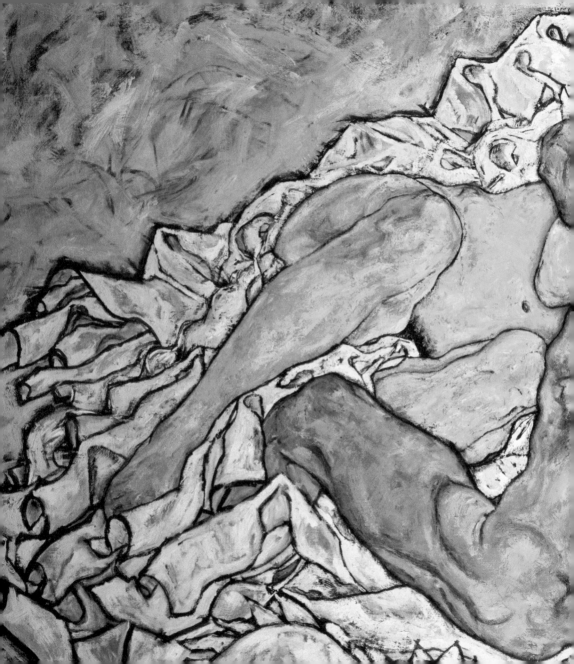

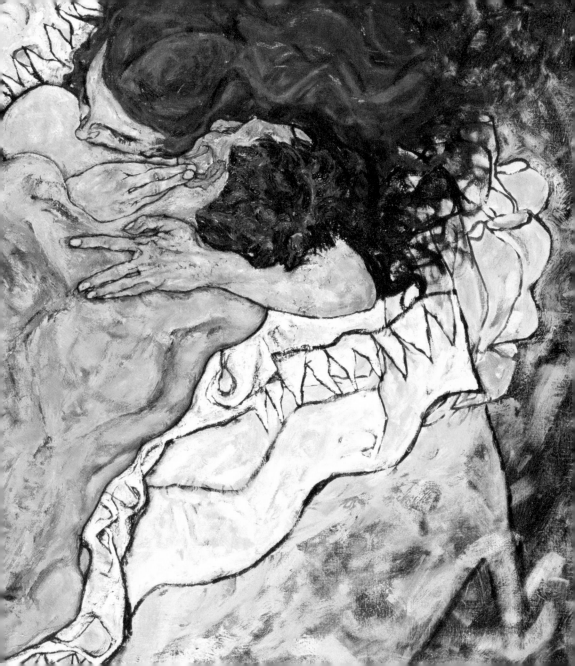

THE ART OF LOVE

by Ovid

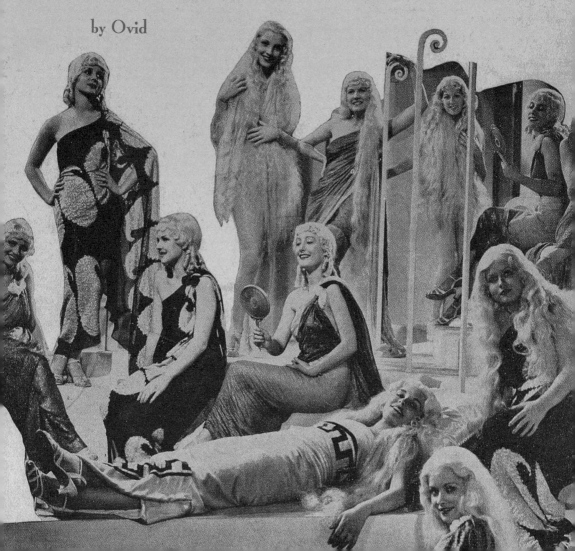

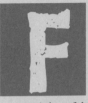irst, consider your appearance. Beauty is a gift of the gods, but only a few receive this gift. Most of you must enhance nature with artful raiment. The rustic carelessness of our forefathers' dress has given way to subtly revealing garments and elaborate adornments. It is not, however, necessary, to drag down your ears with masses of pearls or make walking difficult with the weight of heavy brocades. Moderation, as well as fastidiousness, is more alluring than showiness.

Neither neglect your hair nor depend upon its natural state. It is glamorous only when properly coiffed. There are a thousand ways of dressing the hair, and you must find the one most flattering to you. Your mirror can tell you. If your face is long and oval, part your hair in the middle. If it is round, lengthen it with a topknot. Some women look most charming when they let their hair fall down to their shoulders, like the lyre-playing Apollo; others look best when they bind their tresses tightly like Diana, the chaste huntress. One girl delights us with little curls; another flattens her hair sleekly across the temples. Some women affect high tortoise-shell combs; others crown their heads with towering waves; still others arrange their coiffure in a seemingly casual manner. Real art often seems artless. Think how lucky you are. Sooner or later men grow bald and show their age. Women, however, can disguise age by dyeing their hair—often the artificial color is more attractive than the original shade. Even if your hair should thin, you can always obtain a thick head of hair with a little money.

I should not go into too many intimate details, but I should warn you against the smell of perspiration. Be careful about washing your armpits, and do not let you legs grow unsightly with bristling hairs. You doubtless know how to whiten your skin with powders and redden your cheeks with carmine. You also know how to pencil your eyebrows, widen the space between them, and make your eyes shine brighter by applying saffron to the lids. These things will help cover the marks made by the years.

Avoid the Greek ointments which turn rancid, and be careful of the oils which are extracted from the malodorous fleece of sheep.

There are many things which men need not know about—things which, if seen in their naked reality, would shock them. Observing the lifelike trappings which transform the stage, we do not want to know that they are only props, plain wood tricked out with gilt. The audience is not expected to examine them too closely. In the same way, your private audience should not discover how artificial are your properties.

Most of my pupils are average women. The great beauties need little of my advice, but the plain ones—the great majority—will benefit by it. There are few faces without blemishes—hide the flaws with skill and circumspection. Remedy the defects of your figure. If you are short, sit down most of the time; this way men will not be aware of your lack of height. If you are so small as to be almost a dwarf, lie down and throw something over your feet.

Your voice can be a great lure; sound has as much enticement as sight. Ulysses had to pour wax into the ears of his companions to protect them against the seduction of the sirens' song. You, too, should learn to sing; a thrilling voice may compensate for the lack of other attractions.

When you have got your lover in your net, let him think he is the only one you care to capture. Once, however, you get him in bed, let him suspect a rival. This device always sharpens a man's ardor. A race horse makes better time when several other horses are competing with him rather than when he is running alone. Do not be too obvious about it. Pique him with stories of imaginary lovers; pretend that some man's emissary is always pleading at your door; if you are married, delude him into the belief that your husband is violently jealous and watchfully suspicious. There are times when, though he might enter naturally by the door, you should insist that he creep in stealthily by the window. You might even create a dramatic scene. At the proper moment, have your maid rush in and cry out, "We are discovered!" To make up for such alarms, let there be nights when he has every pleasure without disturbance.

I don't think it's necessary for me to tell a married woman how to deceive her husband. Certainly a wife should respect and fear her spouse—that is the law. But does this mean that she is a slave? If your husband had as many means of watching you as Argus has eyes, you could still outwit him. Can he stop you from writing a letter when you are in your bath? Can he prevent your maid from hiding the note in her bosom or inside her shoe? Lines written in milk are invisible, until read over charcoal. Even if he knows about such tricks, a few words can be scribbled on your maid's body; her flesh will serve as a living tablet.

At a banquet or any other formal meal, be sure to arrive late. Remain dignified and do not carouse until the evening is well advanced; men who have been imbibing freely will find even a plain and modest girl alluring. Eat slowly and with delicacy. Handle the food only with the tips of your fingers. Do not leave greasy marks around your mouth; wipe your hands often. Drink, but only a little. Love and wine are natural companions, but no one likes to see a woman drunk. Don't fall asleep after the meal; a sleeping woman is an open invitation to rape.

I fear to go on, but Venus insists. "That which you hesitate to disclose," she says, "is the most important part of all." So . . . Learn what postures suit you best in the arena of love. If your face is pretty, lie upon your back; if your hips are shapely, show them off. If you are short, be your lover's jockey. If you are tall, kneel. Remember that love has countless ways and poses. ∎

—From *Amores*, first published in 10 BC.

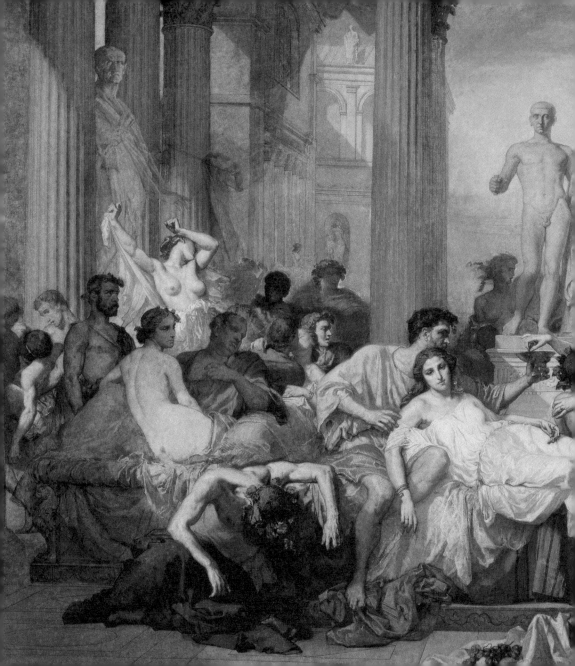

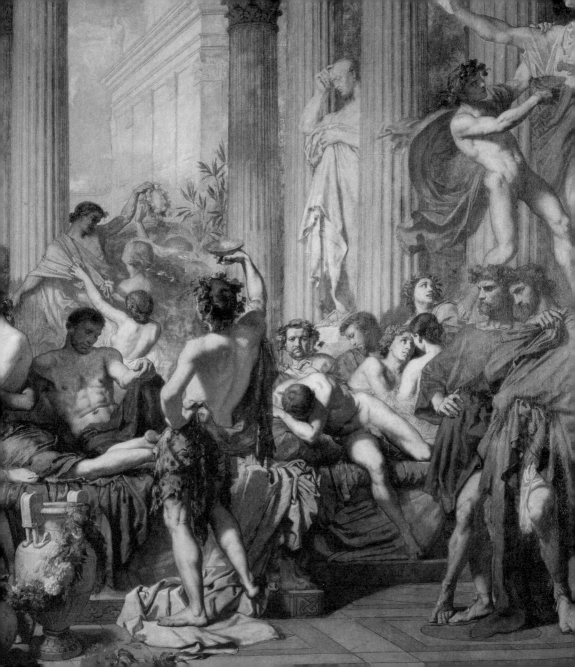

LYSISTRATA

by Aristophanes

Early dawn—Lysistrata walks restlessly up, down and across the stage.
Enter Calonice, Myrrhine, Lampito and others.

LAMPITO: Whose idea was it, to bring us women together this early?

LYSISTRATA: Mine.

LAMPITO: Go on, tell us what's up?

LYSISTRATA: Gladly, my dear. A great deal . . .

MYRRHINE: What's so important? Go on, tell us!

LYSISTRATA: I'll tell you. But first answer one simple question.

MYRRHINE: Out with it!

LYSISTRATA: Don't you miss the fathers of your youngsters? I'll bet anything
that this very moment every one of your husbands is in the army far
away.

CALONICE: Mine has been away five months in Thrace, keeping an eye on
the General.

MYRRHINE: Mine has been away seven long months at Pylus.

LAMPITO: As for mine, whenever he returns home on furlough, he barely
gets inside, but that he pulls out his lance and flies back to the front,
leaving me in the lurch.

CALONICE: Not even the touch of a man for love or money. Ever since
Miletus played us dirty with his leather import restrictions, we can't
find anywhere that eight inch leather toy, the widow's little consoler.

LYSISTRATA: If I find a way to end this war, will you back me up?

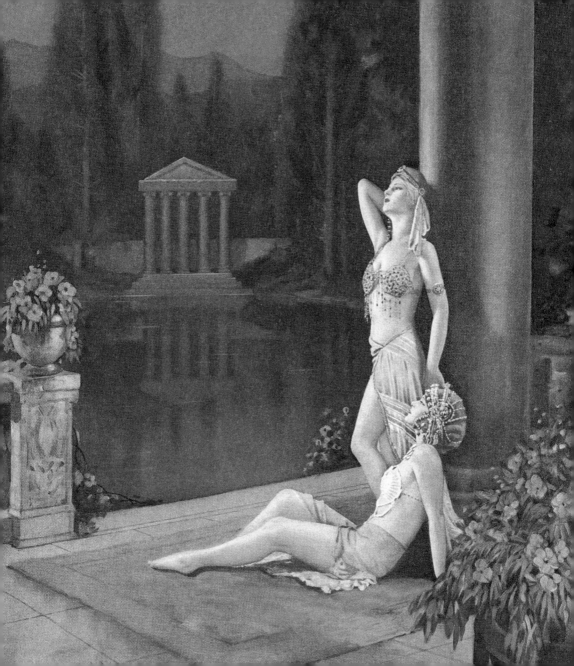

MYRRHINE: I swear I will, even if I have to strip myself and pawn my best dress for this bout . . . *(to the audience)* . . . and drink up the money.

CALONICE: And so will I, though I'm split in my middle like a fish for peace.

LAMPITO: I'd scale the highest mountain bare assed just to get a peep at peace!

LYSISTRATA: Very well then. I'll tell you my plan. If we would force our men to make peace, we must abstain . . .

CALONICE: Abstain from what? Tell us, tell us!

LYSISTRATA: Will you do it?

MYRRHINE: We will, we will! Even if we die for it!

LYSISTRATA: We must abstain from our husbands' arms . . . Yes, we must abstain . . . *(hesitates, then blurts out)* . . . abstain from fucking, absolutely . . . Why do you turn away? Why such sour looks? Where are you going? Why bite your lower lip? Why so pale? Why so dismal? Why the tears? Will you do it? Yes or no? Speak up, say something!

MYRRHINE: No! I can't do without it. Let the war continue . . .

LYSISTRATA: And you, my pretty little fish, you who just now volunteered to be split up the middle for peace?

CALONICE: Anything, anything but this! Ask me to walk through fire . . . but to expect me to give up the sweetest thing in the world, dear, dear Lysistrata! Never!

LYSISTRATA: And you?

ISMANIA: I agree with her. I'd rather be burned alive.

LYSISTRATA: Oh, how weak and lecherous we women are! No wonder Euripides makes tragedies about us. Are we good for nothing but to be fucked and have babies? But you, my dear, you from tough Sparta, if you will stick with me everything may yet be saved. Help me, stick by me, I beg of you Lampito, darling.

LAMPITO: Frankly, it is tough for a woman to sleep without a stiff one pecking in her cage, but Peace at any price!

LYSISTRATA: Oh, my darling, my dearest friend, you are the only real woman here.

CALONICE: But if we, Zeus for bid it, abstain from that swollen, darling thing, will peace come for sure?

LYSISTRATA: Sure, positively sure. Sure as hardness comes, softness follows! All we have to do is to stay home in our best make-up, dressed in our finest translucent silk gowns, nude underneath, with our nests neatly shaved. The sight will make our men's cocks stand like mad and they will be wild to get into us and beg us to spread our thighs. If then we say, "Nothing doing," they will rush to make peace. . . be sure of that.

LAMPITO: Just like Menelaus, who, about to stab his wife, at the sight of her beautiful naked breasts, threw his sword away.

CALONICE: What if they leave us flat?

LYSISTRATA: Then we'll have to find suitable substitutes.

MYRRHINE: Faugh on your substitutions! What if they drag us by force into the bedroom?

LYSISTRATA: Hold on to the door-posts, tight!

CALONICE: What if they beat us, try to rape us?

LYSISTRATA: You'd better give in, but be sulky and nasty about it. Then they won't enjoy it. Men find no pleasure ramming it in by force. Besides, there are a million ways to torment them. Must I teach you how? Don't worry, they will soon give in because there is no fun in it for a man unless the woman waggles merrily along with him.

CALONICE: If you are sure, we'll go along . . .

Several days have passed. Enter Lysistrata, restless.

LYSISTRATA: Quick, quick come here!

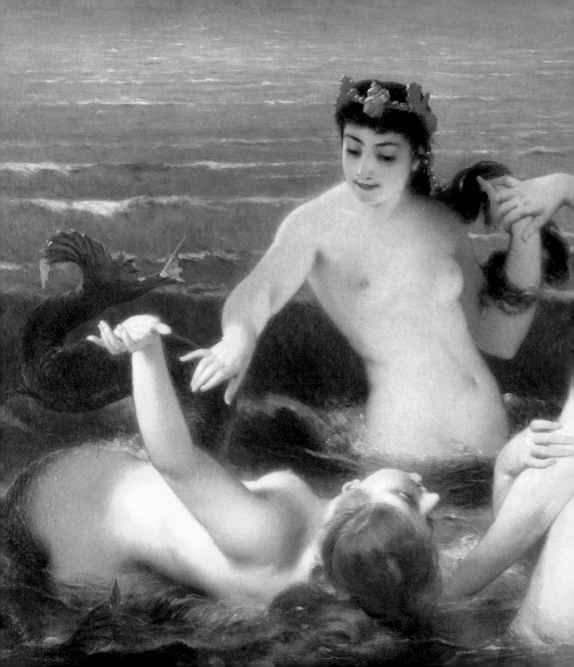

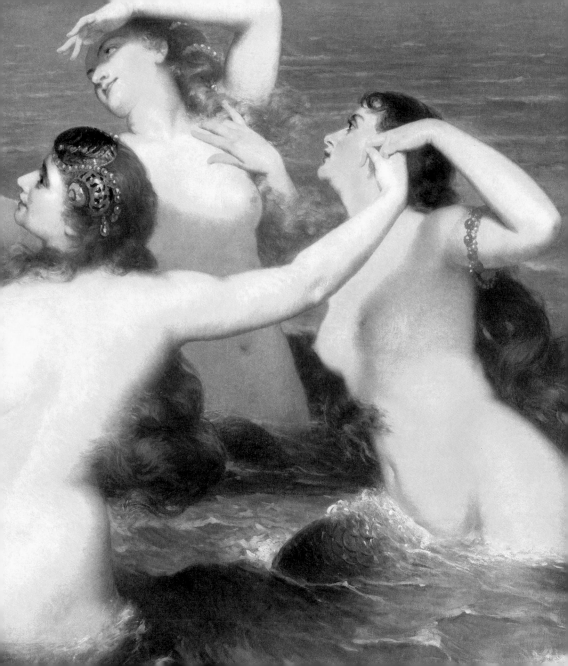

FIRST WOMAN: What is it! What's the matter!

LYSISTRATA: A man! A man! I see a man coming! He is burning up with love's fire. Divine Aphrodite, queen of Cyprus, Paphos and Cythera, I beg you, be kind to our enterprise, keep us firm to our oath!

FIRST WOMAN: A man! Where, where!

LYSISTRATA: There, near the Temple of Chloe.

FIRST WOMAN: Yes, yes I see him! Who is he?

LYSISTRATA: Does anybody recognize him?

MYRRHINE: I do! I do! 'Tis my husband Kinesias. Poor man, how he suffers.

LYSISTRATA: Now to business! It is your job, Myrrhine, to inflame, torment and torture him with love play. Caress him, kiss him, fondle him, cocktease him do everything. Everything except the thing he wants most. That, our oath forbids.

MYRRHINE: Don't worry, I shan't botch the job.

LYSISTRATA: I will stay here and help you keep him hot, make him squirm. You girls to inside.

Enter Kinesias.

KINESIAS: *(to the audience)* See, see how I'm tortured by the spasms . . . This hard-on is killing me!

LYSISTRATA: Ho! Who goes there?

KINESIAS: Me!

LYSISTRATA: What! A man!

KINESIAS: Damn right a man! Can't you see!

LYSISTRATA: Go way! Beat it!

KINESIAS: Who are you to drive me away?

LYSISTRATA: The guard of the day.

KINESIAS: By all the gods, please call Myrrhine!

LYSISTRATA: Call Myrrhine? Why, who are you?

KINESIAS: I'm her loving, suffering husband, Kinesias, son of Peonis.

LYSISTRATA: Ah, good day to you, my friend. Your name is well known to us. Your wife has it on her lips all the time. She never sucks an egg or nibbles a banana without saying, "Just like Kinesias."

KINESIAS: Really! Thank god!

LYSISTRATA: Really, by Aphrodite! And whenever we talk, boasting of our men, your wife quickly says, "Ah, your men! Theirs is nothing compared to my darling's prize winner!"

KINESIAS: I beg of you, please bring her to me.

LYSISTRATA: And what will you give me for my trouble?

KINESIAS: This, if you can stand it . . . *(shaking his erect penis)* . . . I will let you dandle it, if you're game.

LYSISTRATA: My, my! I'll go and fetch her for you.

KINESIAS: Hurry, hurry! Life has no meaning for me since she's gone. I am exhausted carrying around this useless lance. When I got home, I found the house empty, cold. The food is tasteless. And all this while my flaming torch is burning me up.

MYRRHINE: I love him! How I love him! But he doesn't really want me . . . No, I shall not come!

KINESIAS: I beg you, sweetheart. Please, darling.

MYRRHINE: Why do you beg? You really don't want me.

KINESIAS: What, I don't want you! Look, see how stiff my cock stands for you only!

MYRRHINE: Good-bye, my love!

KINESIAS: *(to the audience)* My god, how beautiful she is, and younger looking, too! How lovingly she looks at me. Her disdain only makes me hotter! *(to Myrrhine)* You were foolish, my sweet, to let yourself be led astray by the nasty women. Why cause me such heartaches, suffering, and yourself . . . Your thing and mine down there are going to ruin . . .

MYRRHINE: Keep your hands to yourself, sir!

KINESIAS: Everything is going to the dogs at home . . .

MYRRHINE: I don't care—you sir, stop patting my bottom . . .

KINESIAS: But the cocks and hens are pecking your precious webs to pieces . . . don't you care?

MYRRHINE: Very little. Sir, you better stop groping at once! I'm going . . .

KINESIAS: Don't darling, don't go! We haven't observed the rites of Aphrodite for seven long months . . . Oh, won't you darling, sweet little cunt, perform then now?

MYRRHINE: No, not 'til you men sign a treaty ending the war . . . meanwhile, keep your fingers to yourself, you darling bastard!

KINESIAS: Well, if it's so damned important to you, why, we'll make it, your treaty.

MYRRHINE: That's fine. Soon as you do that, I'll come home, my darling, my stiff one. 'Til then, I swore I'd stay here. Now, no more of this kind of foolishness. Keep your hands to yourself, you . . .

KINESIAS: At least let's have a fast one, my beautiful . . .

MYRRHINE: No! No! How I love you and want you. Keep away!

KINESIAS: But darling, if you love me, why refuse me, my sweet, my little cunt! Let's have a fast one right now . . .

MYRRHINE: It'll be fast enough, I'm sure.

KINESIAS: There's nothing to stop us. Let's get going, come!

MYRRHINE: You poor suffering man, where, where shall we do it?

KINESIAS: In the cave of Pan, there's nothing better.

MYRRHINE: But where will I douche and purify myself before going back to the temple?

KINESIAS: Nothing easier. You can bathe yourself in the spring near the Acropolis.

MYRRHINE: But my oath? Do you want me to break it?

KINESIAS: I'll take all responsibility, don't you worry. I'll say I forced you.

MYRRHINE: Well, all right. I'll go and find a bed . . . meanwhile, keep it up.

KINESIAS: Oh, don't bother, darling. Let's do it on the ground . . .

MYRRHINE: No, you naughty man, you! I couldn't stand you lying on the rocky ground bare assed . . . you just keep it up until I return. *(she runs out)*

KINESIAS: Ah, how the dear girl loves me!

MYRRHINE: *(returning with a cot)* Come, get to bed, quick! I'll undress at once. But dammit, we must have a mattress.

KINESIAS: A mattress! Oh, no! Come here, my juicy one!

MYRRHINE: No, by Artemis. Lie on that rough sacking! Never! That's too dirty, too mean. I'm no whore!

KINESIAS: Please, darling, let me kiss . . .

MYRRHINE: *(she laughs and gives him a kiss)* There, dear! *(she runs out)*

KINESIAS: For heaven's sake, come back quick.

MYRRHINE: *(returning with a mattress)* Here's a mattress . . . You lie down. I'll undress now . . . But, by Aphrodite, we have no pillow . . .

KINESIAS: I don't want a pillow. I want you . . .

MYRRHINE: But I do . . . right under you . . . *(she runs out)*

KINESIAS: Darling, darling why prolong my agony!

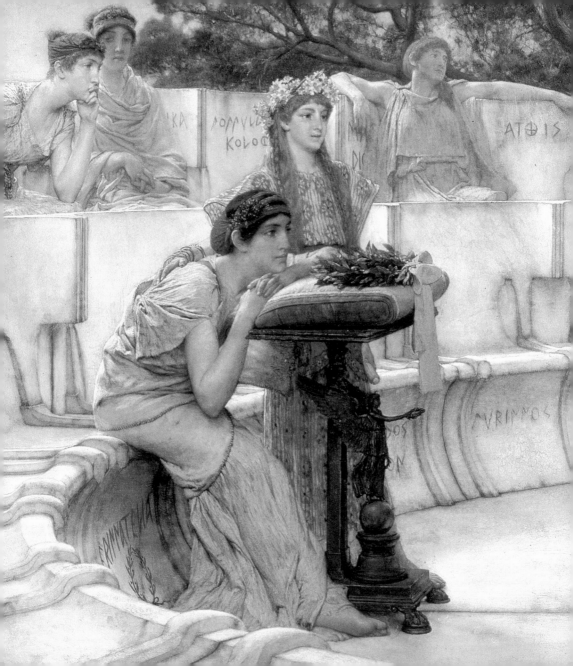

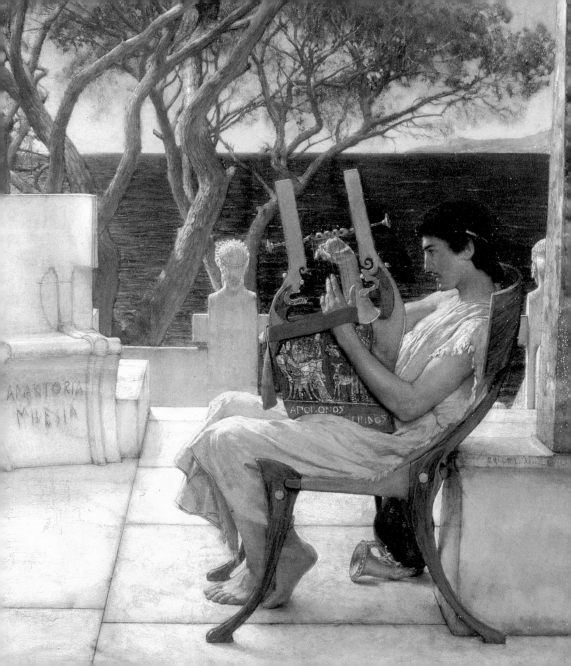

MYRRHINE: *(returning with a pillow)* There, lift your back, dear!

KINESIAS: Got everything now?

MYRRHINE: Let's see, is it everything?

KINESIAS: Come, come, my love, my sweet jewel box . . .

MYRRHINE: I'm just taking off my girdle. But don't forget what you promised me . . . PEACE! Mind you, you keep your word.

KINESIAS: Yes, yes, I sure will! Anything you want! May I die if I don't . . .

MYRRHINE: What, my dear, you have no blanket . . .

KINESIAS: Great Zeus! I don't want a blanket. All I want for a cover is your hot, nibbling cunt . . . Let's get going . . .

MYRRHINE: Take it easy, we'll get there. I'll hurry back in no time flat! *(she rushes out)*

KINESIAS: The darling woman will kill me with her beds, her mattresses, her blankets.

MYRRHINE: *(returning with a blanket)* Now, dear, get up for a second.

KINESIAS: See, I've been up for hours . . . and ready!

MYRRHINE: Would you like me to rub you down with some perfume?

KINESIAS: No, please sweetheart, no!

MYRRHINE: By Aphrodite, I will! You'll smell real sweet. *(she runs out)*

KINESIAS: Damn it! We'll never get going . . . Perfume, no less!

MYRRHINE: *(returning with bottle)* Here, hold out your hand, rub it in. I'll rub your back . . .

KINESIAS: Phew, I don't like the smell of this stuff! Perhaps it will smell better if I rub it in well. It sure isn't violets!

MYRRHINE: Oh, stupid me! I've brought you the wrong bottle.

KINESIAS: It's good enough, darling. I got the right one here! Let's get going.

MYRRHINE: You must be joking, surely! *(she runs out)*

KINESIAS: To hell with the man who invented perfume!

MYRRHINE: *(returning with bottle)* Here, take this bottle, my Joy!

KINESIAS: I have a better one here, for you, darling. Come, you little, tight cunt, come to bed! No more bringings . . .

MYRRHINE: Coming, I'm coming! Just slipping off my slippers. You dear darling boy, you will vote for peace?

KINESIAS: I'll think it over . . . *(Myrrhine runs away)* . . . I'm a dead man. She's killing me. She's gone and left me standing! Oh, the most beautiful woman has cock-teased me. I must get someone to fuck! You poor little fellow, how can I give you what you want so badly. To Doctor Comfort, he'll get a masseur for you.

Enter Chorus of Old Men

CHORUS OF OLD MEN: Poor miserable man, cock-teased by his own wife! How you must suffer. How I pity you . . . How can any man's back and balls stand such strain? His cock is stiff and rigid and not an open-thighed wench to help him!

KINESIAS: Ye gods, how it hurts! What pains! I can hardly stand it!

CHORUS OF OLD MEN: It is doing of that abandoned slut, your wife.

KINESIAS: No, no! Say she's the sweetest, dearest, most delicious darling.

CHORUS OF OLD MEN: She, the cockteaser, a dearest darling! No, no! She's a hussy, a slut!

KINESIAS: Zeus, god of the heavens and thunder, let loose a tornado to sweep her up in the air, whirling round and round 'til her thighs spread out like eagles' wings, then drop her cunt-down, spinning like a top, around my stiff, burning cock!

Exit all

—Excerpted from the 1968 translation by Jack Brussel from the original comedy wirtten in 411 BC.

Lilian

Alfred, Lord Tennyson, c. 1830

Airy, Fairy Lilian,
Flitting, fairy Lilian,
When I ask her if she love me,
Claps her tiny hands above me,
Laughing all she can;
She 'll not tell me if she love me,
Cruel little Lilian.

When my passion seeks
Pleasance in love-sighs,
She, looking thro' and thro' me
Thoroughly to undo me,
Smiling, never speaks:
So innocent-arch, so cunning-simple,
From beneath her gathered wimple
Glancing with black-bearded eyes,
Till the lightning laughters dimple
The baby-roses in her cheeks;
Then away she flies.

Prythee weep, May Lilian!
Gaiety without eclipse
Whearieth me, May Lilian;
Thro' my every heart it thrilleth
When from crimson-threaded lips
Silver-treble laughter trilleth:
Prythee weep, May Lilian!

Praying all I can,
If prayers will not hush thee,
Airy Lilian,
Like a rose-leaf I will crush thee,
Fairy Lilian.

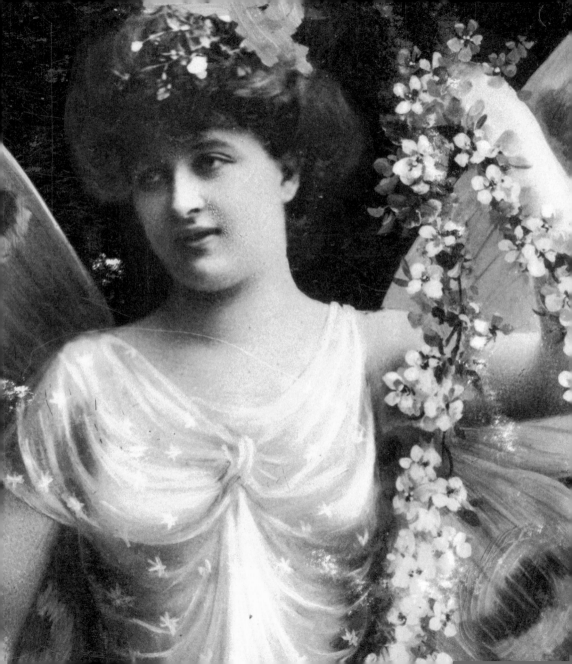

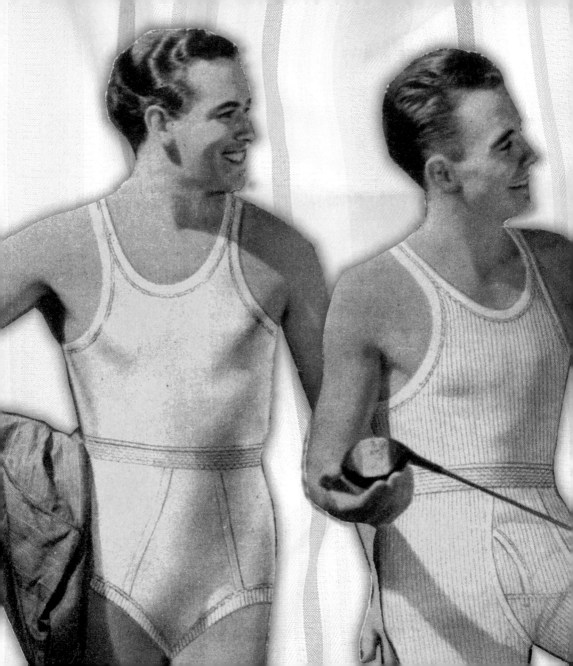

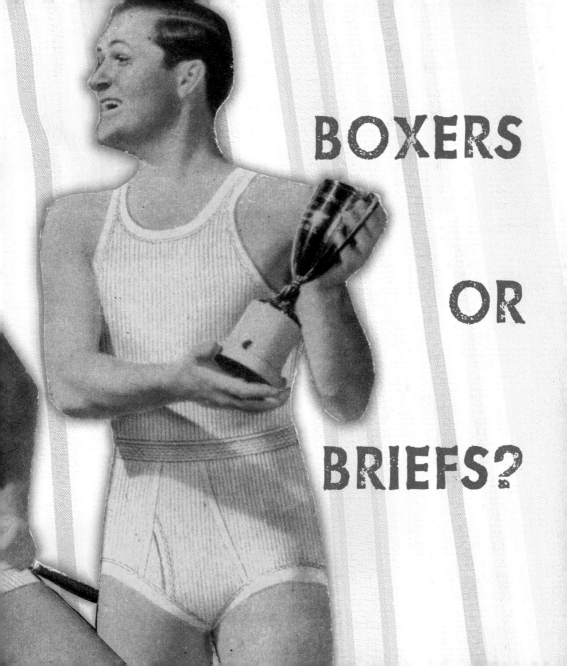

BOXERS

OR

BRIEFS?

ARTHUR SNATCHFOLD

by E. M. Forster

*Sir Richard Conway is staying at the home of a boring
business acquaintance, Trevor Donaldson.*

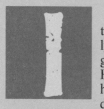

It was a silent sunless morning, and seemed earlier than it actually was. The green of the garden and of the trees was filmed with grey, as if it wanted wiping. Presently the electric pump started. He looked at his watch again, slipped down the stairs, out of the house, across the amphitheatre and through the yew hedge. He did not run, in case he was seen and had to explain. He moved at the maximum pace possible for a gentleman, known to be an original, who fancies an early stroll in his pyjamas. 'I thought I'd have a look at your formal garden, there wouldn't have been time after breakfast' would have been the line. He had of course looked at it the day before, also at the wood. The wood lay before him now, and the sun was just tipping into it. There were two paths through the bracken, a broad and a narrow. He waited until he heard the milk-can approaching down the narrow path. Then he moved quickly, and they met, well out of sight of the Donaldsonian demesne.

"Hullo!" he called in his easy out-of-doors voice; he had several voices, and knew by instinct which was wanted.

"Hullo! Somebody's out early!"

"You're early yourself."

"Me? Whor'd the milk be if I worn't?" the milkman grinned, throwing his head back and coming to a standstill. Seen at close quarters he was coarse, very much of the people and of the thick-fingered earth; a hundred years ago his type was trodden into the mud, now it burst and flowered and didn't care a damn.

"You're the morning delivery, eh?"

"Looks like it." He evidently proposed to be facetious—the clumsy fun which can be so delightful when it falls from the proper lips. "I'm not the evening delivery anyway, and I'm not the butcher nor the grocer, nor'm I the coals."

"Live around here?"

"Maybe. Maybe I don't. Maybe I flop about in them planes."

"You live around here, I bet."

"What if I do?"

"If you do you do. And if I don't I don't."

This fatuous retort was a success, and was greeted with doubled-up laughter. "If you don't you don't! Walking about in yer night things, too, you'll ketch a cold you will, that'll be the end of you! Stopping back in the 'otel, I suppose?"

"No. Donaldson's. You saw me there yesterday."

"Oh, Donaldson's, that's it. You was the old granfa' at the upstairs window."

"Old granfa' indeed . . . I'll granfa' you," and he tweaked at the impudent nose. It dodged, it seemed used to this sort of thing. There was probably nothing the lad wouldn't consent to if properly handled, partly out of mischief, partly to oblige. "Oh, by the way . . ." and he felt the shirt as if interested in the quality of its material. "What was I going to say?" and he gave the zip at the throat a downward pull. Much slid into view. "Oh, I know—when's this round of yours over?"

"'Bout eleven. Why?"

"Why not?"

"'Bout eleven *at*

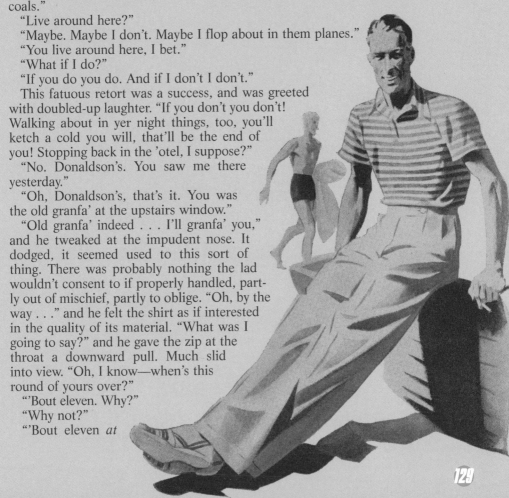

night. Ha ha. Got yer there. Eleven at night. What you want to arst all them questions for? We're strangers, aren't we?"

"How old are you?"

"Ninety, same as yourself."

"What's your address?"

"There you go on! Hi! I like that. Arstin questions after I tell you no."

"Got a girl? Ever heard of a pint? Ever heard of two?"

"Go on. Get out." But he suffered his forearm to be worked between massaging fingers, and he set down his milk-can. He was amused. He was charmed. He was hooked, and a touch would land him.

"You look like a boy who looks all right," the elder man breathed.

"Oh, *stop* it . . . All right, I'll go with you."

Conway was entranced. Thus, exactly thus, should the smaller pleasures of life be approached. They understood one another with a precision impossible for lovers. He laid his face on the warm skin over the clavicle, hands nudged him behind, and presently the sensation for which he had planned so cleverly was over. It was part of the past. It had fallen like a flower upon similar flowers.

He heard "You all right?" It was over there too, part of a different past. They were lying deeper in the wood, where the fern was highest. He did not reply, for it was pleasant to lie stretched thus and to gaze up through bracken fronds at the distant treetops and the pale blue sky, and feel the exquisite pleasure fade.

"That was what you wanted, wasn't it?" Propped on his elbows the young man looked down anxiously. All his roughness and pertness had gone, and he only wanted to know whether he had been a success.

"Yes . . . Lovely."

"Lovely? You say lovely?" he beamed, prodding gently with his stomach.

"Nice boy, nice shirt, nice everything."

"That a fact?"

Conway guessed that he was vain, the better sort often are, and laid on the flattery thick to please him, praised his comeliness, his thrusting

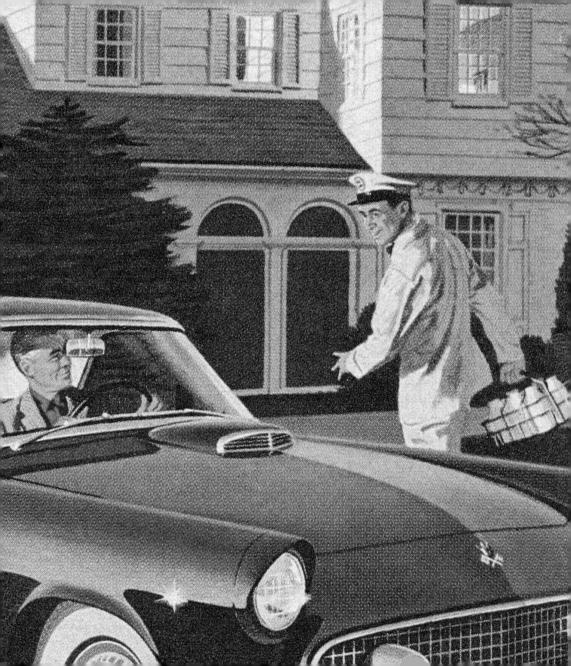

thrashing strength; there was plenty to praise. He liked to do this and to see the broad face grinning and feel the heavy body on him. There was no cynicism in the flattery, he was genuinely admiring and gratified.

"So you enjoyed that?"

"Who wouldn't?"

"Pity you didn't tell me yesterday."

"I didn't know how to."

"I'd a met you down where I have my swim. You could 'elped me strip, you'd like that. Still, we mustn't grumble." He gave Conway a hand and pulled him up, and brushed and tidied the raincoat like an old friend. "We could get seven years for this, couldn't we?"

"Not seven years, still we'd get something nasty. Madness, isn't it? What can it matter to anyone else if you and I don't mind?"

"Oh, I suppose they've to occupy themselves with somethink or other," and he took up the milk-can to go on.

"Half a minute, boy—do take this and get yourself some trifle with it." He produced a note which he had brought on the chance.

"I didn't do it fer that."

"I know you didn't."

"Naow, we was each as bad as the other . . . Naow . . . keep yer money."

"I'd be pleased if you would take it. I expect I'm better off than you and it might come in useful. To take out your girl, say, or towards your next new suit. However, please yourself, of course."

"Can you honestly afford it?"

"Honestly."

"Well, I'll find a way to spend it, no doubt. People don't always behave as nice as you, you know."

Conway could have returned the compliment. The affair had been trivial and crude, and yet they both had behaved perfectly. They would never meet again, and they did not exchange names. After a hearty handshake, the young man swung away down the path, the sunlight and shadow rushing over his back. He did not turn around, but his arm, jerking sideways to

balance him, waved an acceptable farewell. The green
flowed over his brightness, the path bent, he disap-
peared. Back he went to his own life, and through the
quiet of the morning his laugh could be heard as he
whooped at the maids.

Conway waited for a few
moments, as arranged, and then he
went back too. His luck held. He
met no one, either in the amphitheatre garden or on the stairs, and after
he had been in his room for a minute
the maid arrived with his early tea. "I'm
sorry the milk was late again, sir," she
said. He enjoyed it, bathed and shaved
and dressed himself for town. It was the
figure of a superior city-man which was
reflected in the mirror as he tripped downstairs. The car came round after breakfast to
take him to the station, and he was completely sincere when he told the Trevor
Donaldsons that he had had an out-of-the-
way pleasant weekend. They believed him,
and their faces grew brighter. "Come again
then, come by all means again," they cried
as he slid off. In the train he read the
papers rather less than usual and smiled
to himself rather more. It was so pleasant
to have been completely right over a
stranger, even down to little details like
the texture of the skin. It flattered his
vanity. It increased his sense of power. ■

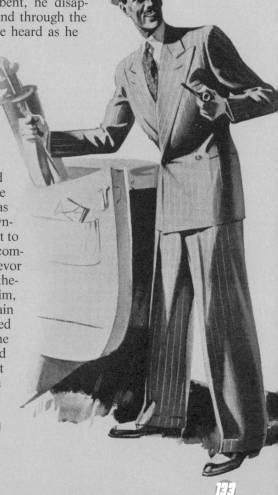

—From "Arthur Snatchfold," a short story written in 1928.

I LIKE MY BEER COLD, MY TV LOUD AND MY HOMOSEXUALS FLAMING.

—HOMER SIMPSON

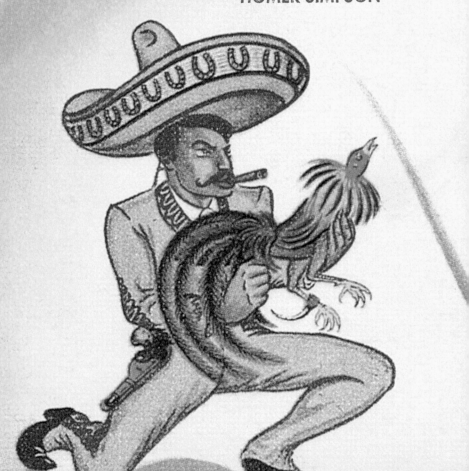

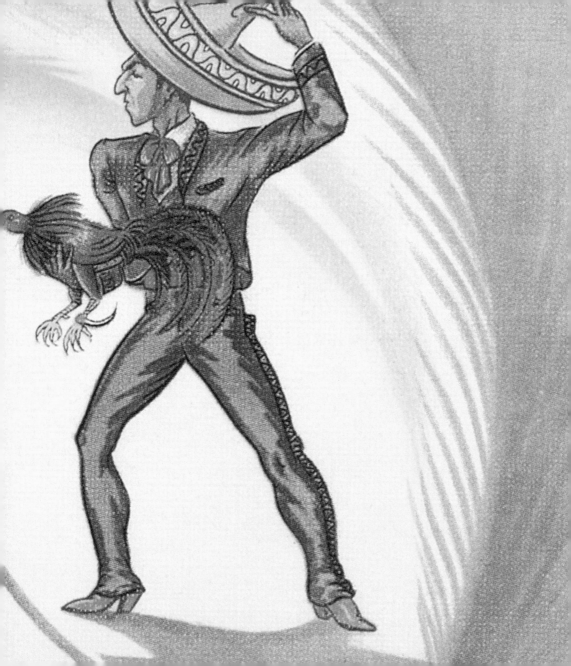

GA

JOHN

Texas

VEGETA

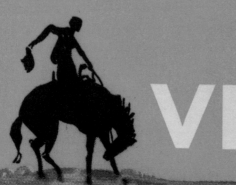

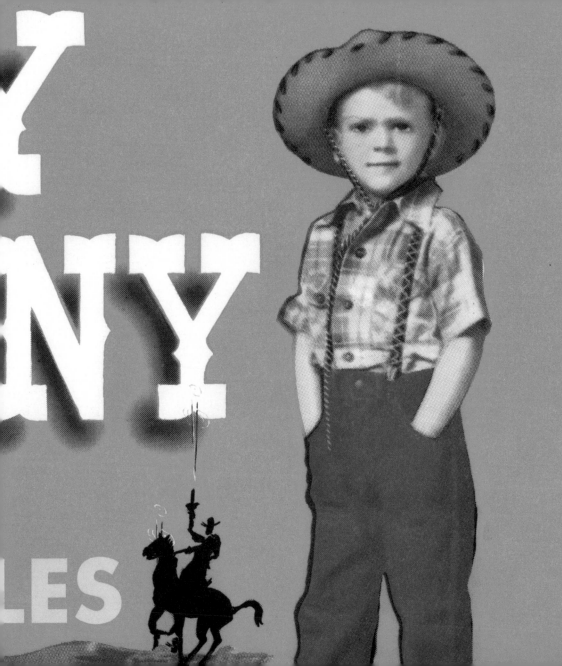

The Hanky Code

The handkerchief code—seldom used today—became a popular way to get your preferences across in gay bars of the 1970s. Placing a certain colored hanky in the appropriate rear pocket (see chart) instantly advertised your interests. The hankies could also be mixed and matched so if, for example, you saw apricot, brown-and-white striped, chamois and paisley hankies tied around a teddy bear sticking out of someone's left back pocket you were clearly looking at a chubby biker wearing boxer shorts looking for a cuddle with a latino.

COMMON

Worn on Left	Color	Worn on Right
Heavy S&M Top	Black	Heavy S&M Bottom
Bondage Top	Grey	Bondage Bottom
Golden Shower Top	Yellow	Golden Shower Bottom
Piercer	Purple	Piercee
Top	Dark Blue	Bottom
Wants Oral Sex	Light Blue	Expert at Oral Sex
Likes Drag	Lavender	In Drag
Uniform Top	Olive Drab	Uniform Bottom

UNCOMMON

Worn on Left	Color	Worn on Right
Sixty-niner	Robin's Egg Blue	Sixty-niner
Likes Navel Worship	Mauve	Navel Worshipper
Has 8" or More	Mustard	Size Queen
Rides a Motorcycle	Chamois	Likes Bikers
2 Looking for 1	Gold	1 Looking for 2
Anything Goes	Orange	Not Now, Thanks
Two Tons O'Fun	Apricot	Chubby Chaser
Foot Fetish Top	Coral	Shrimper
Likes Latino Bottom	Brown & White Stripes	Likes Latino Top
A Cowboy	Rust	His Horse
Wears Boxer Shorts	Paisley	Likes Boxer Shorts
Spanker	Fuschia	Spankee
Cuddler	Teddy Bear	Cuddlee

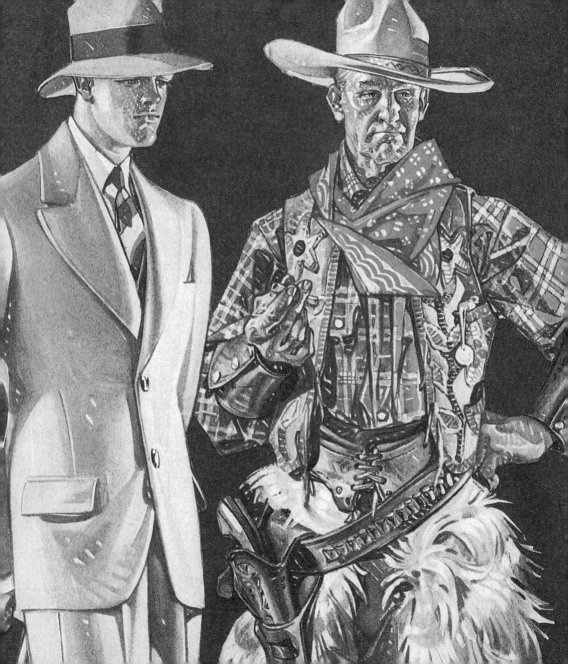

Dr. Kinsey Knocking...

"The only unnatural sex act is that which you cannot perform." So said Dr. Alfred Kinsey, who conducted the first mass scientific survey of human sexual behavior. The results, published in 1948 and 1953, were popularly known as *The Kinsey Reports*. Here are two interviews.

FEMALE, age 54, divorced at age 39

Q. Have you ever paid a male for intercourse?
A. *Yes, I have.*

Q. How young were you the first time you ever paid a male for intercourse?
A. *I was 43.*

Q. And when was the last time you paid a man?
A. *Just last year.*

Q. Between the ages of 43 to 53, how often did you pay for intercourse?
A. *Oh, I used such services quite regularly.*

Q. How regularly would you say?
A. *I can't really remember precisely.*

Q. Was it every week, or twice a year, or once a month?
A. *I started with one gentleman on a regular basis for the first six years.*

Q. How regularly did you see him during that period?
A. *I saw him about twice a month.*

Q. Did you pay anyone else for intercourse during those first six years, say from age 43 to 49?
A. *No, he was the extent of my interest.*

Q. And from age 49 to 53, how often did you pay for coitus?
A. *Oh, that's easy. I only saw two other men I paid, each one one time only.*

Q. Then you paid for intercourse approximately 146 times, that is twice a month for six years is 144 plus the two single experiences?
A. *I didn't realize it was that much, but the calculations are correct.*

Q. What is the total number of different males you've paid for intercourse?
A. *Well, there was my regular partner of six years and then two others.*

Q. That's right. What were their ages?
A. *Now?*

Q. No, at the time you were having intercourse with them.
A. *Let's see. One was 28, one was about 23 and the other I'm guessing was*

Oh! Dr. Kinsey!

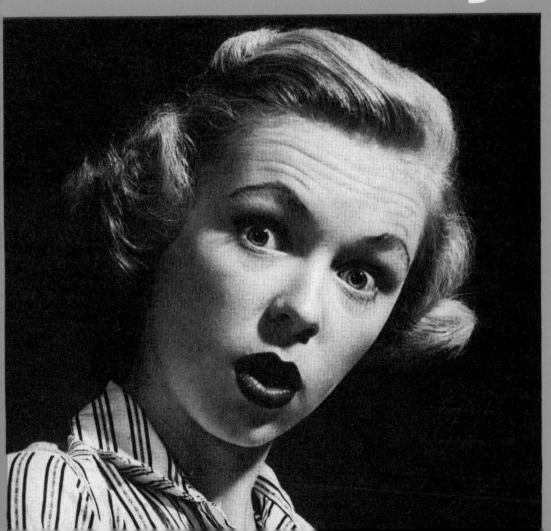

probably somewhere in between, maybe around 26.

Q. How much did you pay the men for intercourse?

A. *You mean including gifts?*

Q. I mean cash on the barrelhead each time you had intercourse.

A. *My regular man was always $100. And the other two were less.*

Q. How much were they?

A. *One was $50 and the other about $35.*

Q. What techniques did you use?

A. *Oh, we just had sex.*

Q. You mean intercourse?

A. *Yes.*

Q. Was there any mouth genital contact?

A. *No. I never allowed that.*

Q. Was there any anal intercourse?

A. *Once, but we always had straight sex.*

Q. Have you ever been paid for intercourse?

A. *Well, it's funny that you should ask. One time I was in a singles bar, and a man insisted on paying me $40 for intercourse, which I would've been happy to have had without payment, but he went ahead and paid me.*

Q. What other times?

A. *That was the only time.*

MALE, eighth-grade education, age 43

Q. How tall are you?

A. *I'm 6 feet tall.*

Q. How much do you weigh?

A. *I weigh 160 lbs.*

Q. What's the most you ever weighed in your life?

A. *Uh, 200 lbs.*

Q. How old were you then?

A. *I was in the Army.*

Q. Well that made you about 20.

A. *Yeah, that's right.*

Q. When your penis is soft, how long would you guess it is?

A. *Oh, it ain't more than 4 inches.*

Q. How long is your penis when it's hard?

A. *I don't know, I never measured it.*

Q. Well, make a guess. Would you say it's this long, this long, or this long? (Interviewer demonstrates possible length, with his or her hands.)

A. *About 6 inches.*

Q. Have you ever been circumcised? Have you ever had skin cut away from the head of your penis?

A. *No, I guess I never did.*

Q. When your penis is hard, do you

have any trouble pulling the skin back over the head?

A. *No, no trouble.*

Q. Is the opening on your penis about here on the tip end or underneath?

A. *No, it's right there on the tip end.*

Q. Do you have two balls?

A. *Uh, yeah.*

Q. Does one hang lower than the other?

A. *Uh, I guess the left one does.*

Q. Would you want to change your body in any way at all? Is there any way you would change it?

A. *Oh, I guess I like my body pretty well.*

Q. Is there anything about your sex partner you'd like to change? Anything about her body?

A. *Well, she weighs about 30 pounds more than I'd like her to weigh, but outside of that, she's a pretty good-looking broad.*

Q. How do you think your sex partner feels about your body?

A. *She don't care.*

Q. What kinds of things do you like in a sex partner?

A. *I like 'em tall, redhead, good teeth, fun loving, and pretty smelling.*

Q. Fine. Anything else?

A. *Yeah, big tits.*

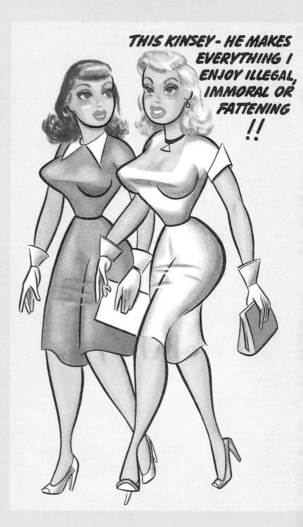

THIS KINSEY – HE MAKES EVERYTHING I ENJOY ILLEGAL, IMMORAL OR FATTENING !!

PRIAPUS WAS HERE!

By the end of the day—August 24, 79 AD—Pompeii, the frisky Roman's playground, was completely buried in volcanic ash. Sixteen hundred years later an architect accidentally came across the ruins and dug up some of the well-preserved and quite-steamy frescoes giving us a peek at the goings-on in ancient Rome. But because times had become much more prudish, some of the images—including one of the uber-male god Priapus—were plastered over and not seen again until 1998.

Beside the lickerish illustrations there were also sculptures, mosaics and even graffiti found giving us more details of life in Pompeii. "If anyone is looking for some tender love in this town, keep in mind that here all the girls are very friendly," is written on the wall of the basilica. Elsewhere a pricelist shows that Athenais cost 2 As, the house slave Logas was 8 and as for Martimus, well, he would "lick your vulva for 4 As," and was "ready to serve virgins as well."

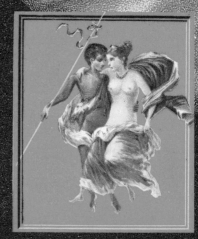

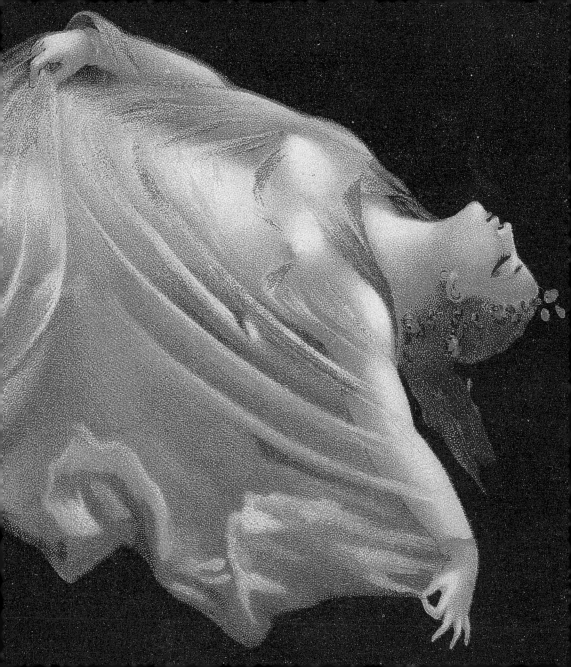

Paraphilia A to Z

ALGOLAGNIA: Deriving sexual pleasure from physical pain

AMAUROPHILIA: Preference for sex with the blind or blindfolded

AQUAPHILIA: Images of people underwater and sex underwater

AUTOGYNEPHILIA: A man's tendency to be sexually aroused by the image of himself as a woman

BALLOON FETISHISM: A fascination with balloons which can involve inflation, popping or simply the movement of the balloon

CELEBRIPHILIA: The obsession to have sex with a celebrity

CRUSH FETISH: The desire to see others crush food, toys or small creatures like insects

FAUNOIPHILIA: Sexual arousal from watching animals have sex

FRUIT FETISH: The use of fruit or vegetables for sexual gratification

HARPAXOPHILIA: Sexual arousal brought about by being robbed

HYBRISTOPHILIA: An attraction to those who have committed cruel or outrageous crimes

INFANTILISM: The desire to wear diapers and be treated as a helpless infant

MACROPHILIA: A sexual attraction to large people

MICROPHILIA: The sexual attraction to smaller people or the desire to be miniaturized

PARAPHILIA: non-mainstream sexual practices that describe sexual feelings toward non-sexual objects

PLUSHOPHILIA: A sexual fondness for large soft furry toys

PODOPHILIA (Foot Fetish): A special interest in feet

SPECTROPHILIA: The sexual attraction to ghosts or arousal from images in mirrors

STATUEPHILIA: Sexual attraction to dolls, statues or lifelike mannequins

TECHNOSEXUALITY (Robot Fetish): An attraction to either humanoid or non-humanoid robots (or people acting like them)

TRICHOPHILIA: Sexual attraction to hair or hairstyles

ZOOPHILIA: Sexual attraction to animals

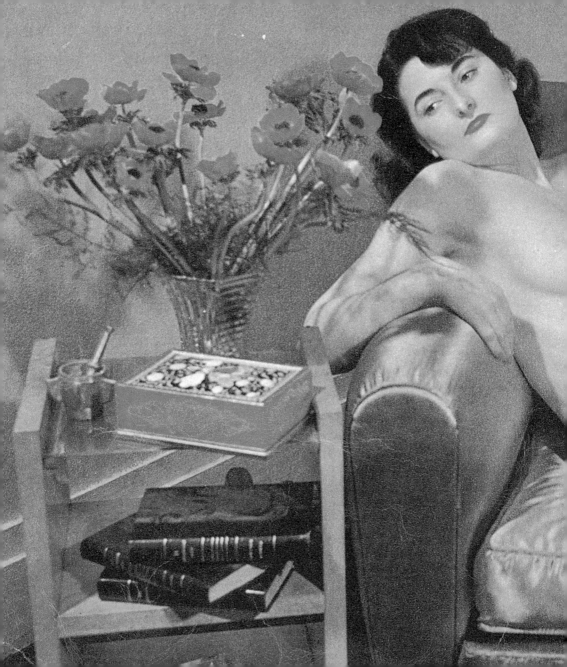

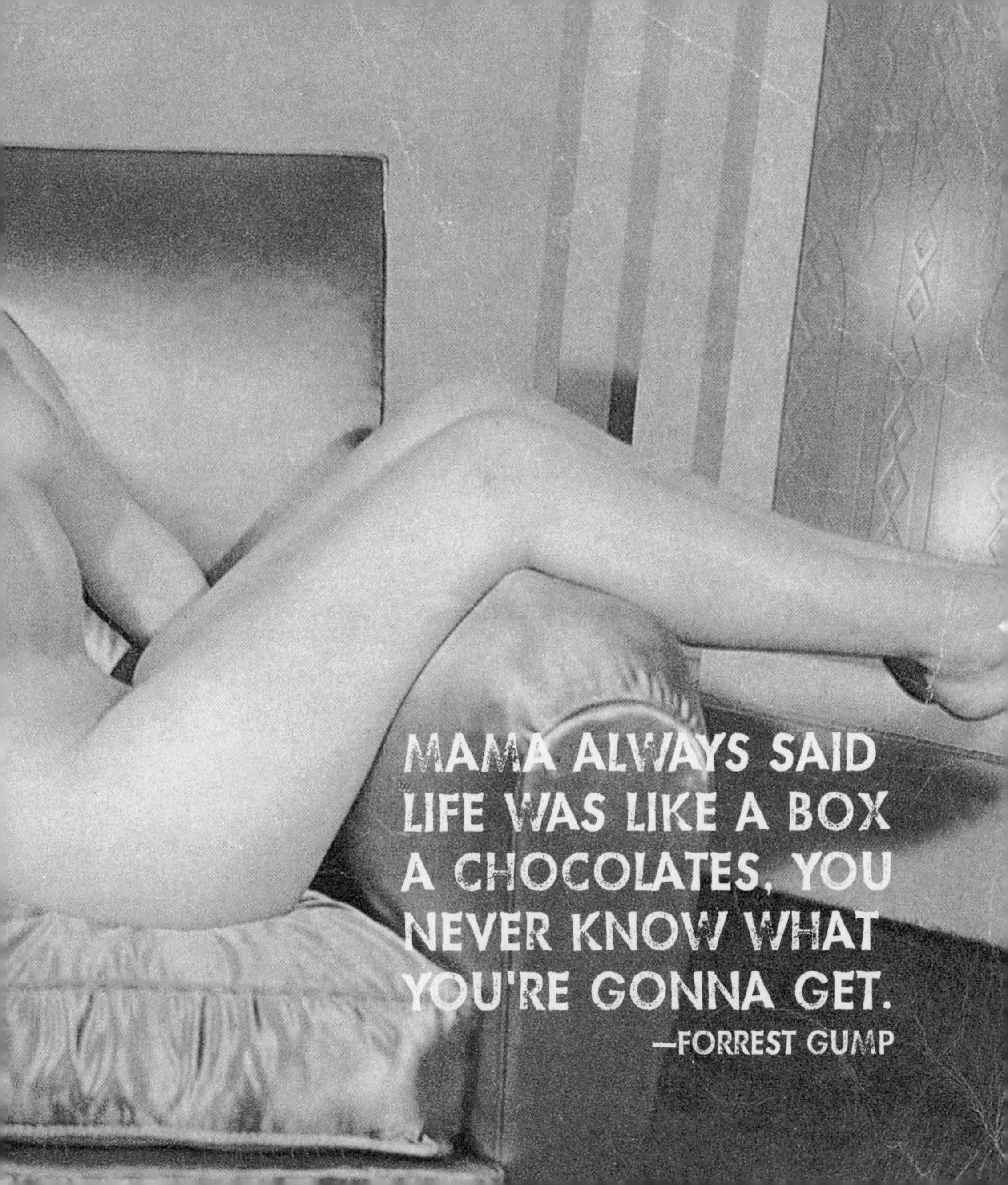

MAMA ALWAYS SAID
LIFE WAS LIKE A BOX
A CHOCOLATES, YOU
NEVER KNOW WHAT
YOU'RE GONNA GET.
—FORREST GUMP

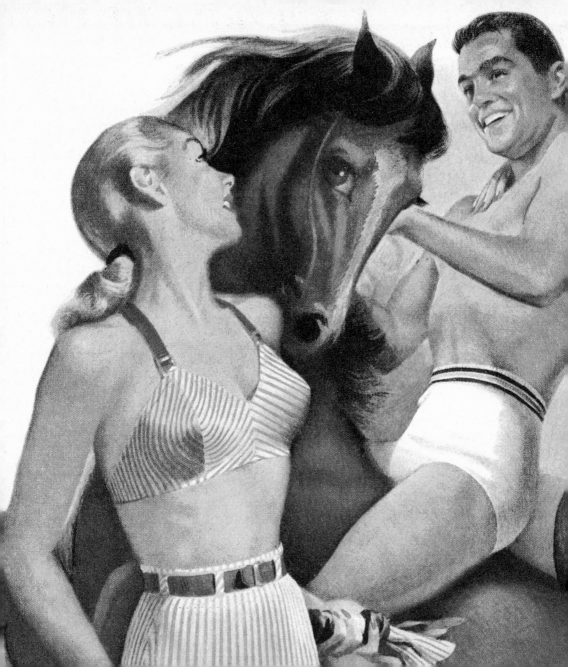

Equus Eroticus

Equus Eroticus is a magazine devoted exclusively to ponygirls and ponyboys—men and women linked together by the desire to use human ponies as an expression of erotic pleasure. . .

"Having one partner assume the role of a human pony while the other partner assumes the Dominant role and controls the role playing scenario of this highly erotic activity, can be a very exciting part of bondage and domination.

Both men and women can play the Dominant or submissive role, and many couples switch roles and develop new ideas as they act out their fantasies.

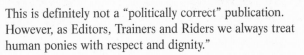

This is definitely not a "politically correct" publication. However, as Editors, Trainers and Riders we always treat human ponies with respect and dignity."

— From the Spring 1997 issue of *Equus Eroticus* (the premiere magazine for the discriminating pony play enthusiast)

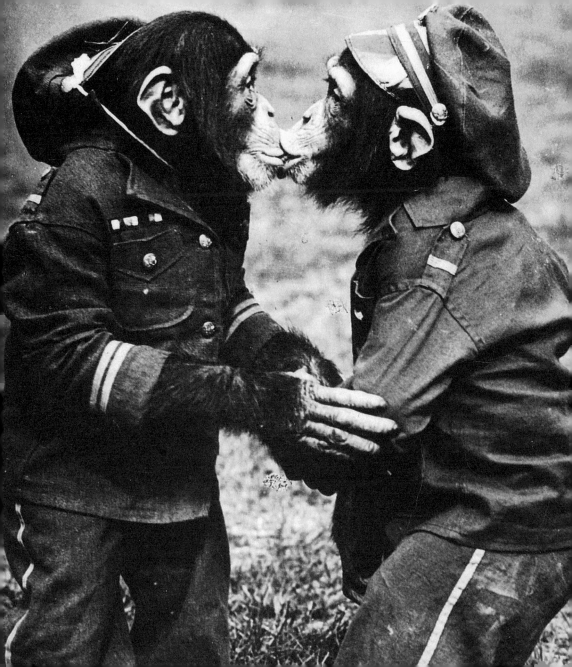

Animal Magnetism

As Cole Porter famously put it, "birds do it, bees do it" . . . but even educated fleas might be surprised to find such diversity in the animal kingdom.

While oysters come in both male and female types, they can morph back and forth several times throughout life.

Porpoises often enjoy group sex.

A humpback whale sports a 10-foot long erection. A Blue whale's testicle can weigh up to 100 pounds.

Male giraffes "neck" for reasons of combat and affection. Amorous males will quite often caress, court, mount and climax. Same-sex relations are, in fact, more frequent than heterosexual behavior.

Lady bedbugs don't come with a vagina. In order to mate the male uses his curved (and tough) penis to literally drill an opening.

The male tick, on the other hand, has no penis at all. He uses his nose to sniff out the female opening, deposits his sperm, then uses his nose to stuff it in.

Human birth control pills work on gorillas.

A pig's orgasm lasts for 30 minutes. A pig's penis is shaped like a corkscrew.

The desert rat can have sex up to 120 times an hour.

During the summer of 2004 over five hundred pigs were ordered killed by the mayor of Nyahururu town, a small village north of Nairobi, Kenya. It seems that the frisky pigs were mating with stray dogs which the mayor claimed "broke the laws of nature and caused unnecessary commotion."

A penguin only has sex twice a year.

Some North American lizard species (*Cnemidophorus uniparens*, for example) are only female. That doesn't stop them from having sex, though. In fact, the sexually active ones produce far more eggs.

Animal Magnetism

Male deer rub their antlers on a tree as a form of masturbation.

Although octopuses face each other when mating, their sex organs never touch. Instead the male squirts onto one of his tentacles then gently places the sperm where it needs to go.

The barnacle has the largest penis of any animal in the world in relation to its size. This is helpful since it's stuck in one spot and uses its instrument to seek out a partner.

In June 2003 the *New York Post* reported (under the heading, "Mother Nature In Manhattan") that aggressive mallards were prowling Central Park. According to the article, these "web-footed fiends" had been attacking unsuspecting American black ducks. The result: a new species dubbed the black duck mallard.

The cicadas' only natural predator is massosporam—a sexually transmitted disease.

Hummingbirds and swifts are truly part of the Mile High Club, often mating while airborne.

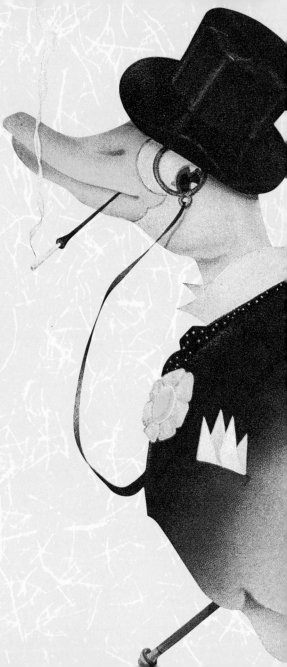

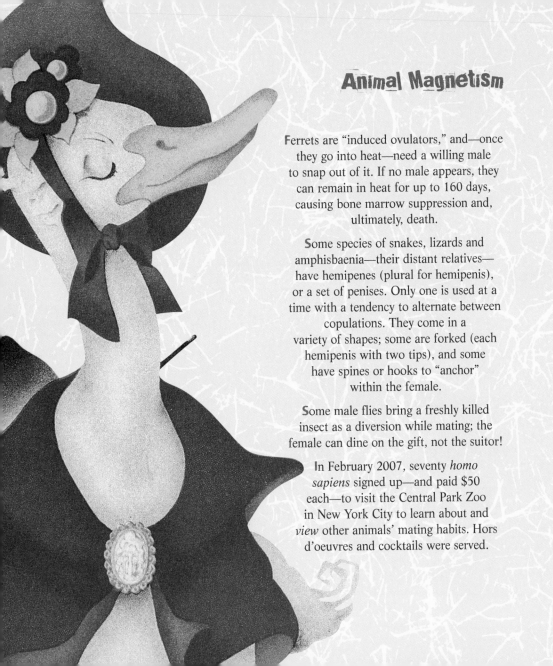

Animal Magnetism

Ferrets are "induced ovulators," and—once they go into heat—need a willing male to snap out of it. If no male appears, they can remain in heat for up to 160 days, causing bone marrow suppression and, ultimately, death.

Some species of snakes, lizards and amphisbaenia—their distant relatives—have hemipenes (plural for hemipenis), or a set of penises. Only one is used at a time with a tendency to alternate between copulations. They come in a variety of shapes; some are forked (each hemipenis with two tips), and some have spines or hooks to "anchor" within the female.

Some male flies bring a freshly killed insect as a diversion while mating; the female can dine on the gift, not the suitor!

In February 2007, seventy *homo sapiens* signed up—and paid $50 each—to visit the Central Park Zoo in New York City to learn about and *view* other animals' mating habits. Hors d'oeuvres and cocktails were served.

PLEASE DON'T BLAME ME

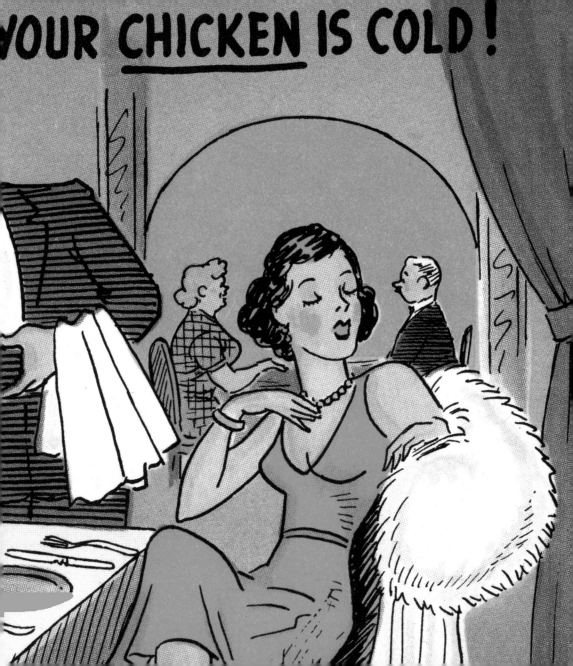

My First Touch of Fur

by Rick Castro

Though "plushie" and "furry" may sound like obscure, specific sorts of fetish, I soon learned that there are sub-fetishes within the scene. On one end are the basic fanboys, who collect furry art. Then there's my personal favorite, plushies. They love inanimate stuffed animals (I don't mean taxidermy, although now I'm convinced this also exists). If they are plushophiles, they love their plush in a more erotic way. Furries walk around wearing cute little ears & tails. I met military furries, sci-fi furries, homosexual zoophiles (who are erotically attracted to real animals), Goth scalies (who love reptiles) and fursuiters.

Some furries are slagged off as "burned fur" because they disapproved of the more yiffy (horny) aspects of the fandom and want the scene to be more "normal." Speaking of normal, people not in the scene are called "mundanes." A mundane might think furry events are thinly veiled versions of bestiality. But that's not so and the B-word is verboten among furries. Although I did meet a few "zoos," this scene is more about fantasy, art and role playing than it is about poking a poodle.

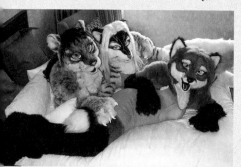

And their artistry would make Disney so jealous, that their "mundane" fur would stand on end.

Furries started as an offshoot of Trekkie conventions. Sometime around 1980, about 20 artists produced *ConFURence 0*. Mucks, or furry chat rooms on the Internet (populated by folks with names like Skunkwiff, Alina Piglet and Marmaduke Master), helped the scene gel and grow to the point where furry events are now held monthly everywhere in the world.

Above: Autumn Fox and friends. Opposite above: Otto in the backyard.

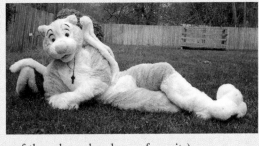

Some fursuits have SPH's, (strategically placed holes) to accommodate relieving and enjoying themselves. They then wear shorts to cover the private holes.

I asked one furry artist named Bushycat why there seemed to be so many gays, transgender and bisexuals in furry fandom. (I always suspect that male bodies are inside some of those hourglass bunny fur suits).

"Sure," she said, "many furries are bi, they're by themselves!"

This catty comment may reek of burned fur, but she was merely being playfully feline. Bushycat is a Rubenesque female furry in her late 20's who wears a faux tiger-fur miniskirt and a plastic Halloween mask that she re-painted to look like a tiger face. I met her at a Seattle furry convention where she displayed her art-work depicting gay male white tigers bound and gagged, spooging with masterful black panthers. She considers her-self a proud and caring cat fag hag.

I discovered through hushed interviews that plushies are the low bears on the totem pole of furry hierarchy. Their cutesy/nerdy demeanors make them prey for the sarcasm of their natural furry predators. "They're just toooo cuddly," one furry sniffed, strictly off the record.

But others I met find the furrydom more welcoming than the outside world. "Before I met the people in the furry world my life was grey," said Alice. "Now it's in living color!"

—Rick Castro is a filmmaker/photographer living in Hollywood, CA. Rick runs and owns the only fetish art gallery in America called, Antebellum Gallery.

159

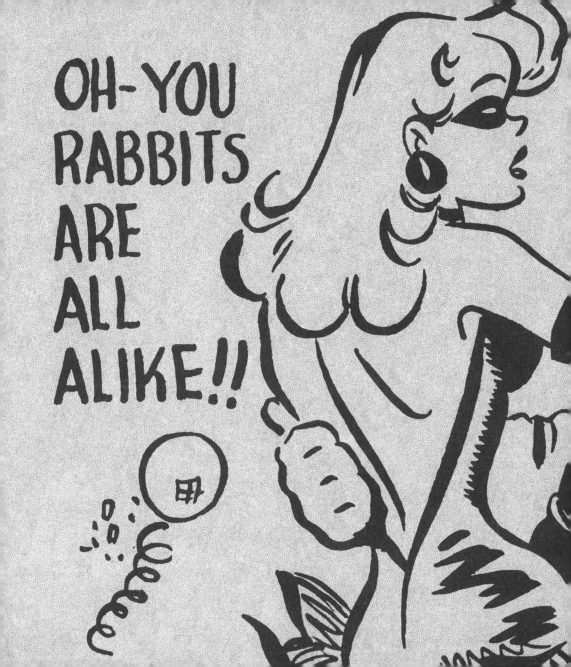

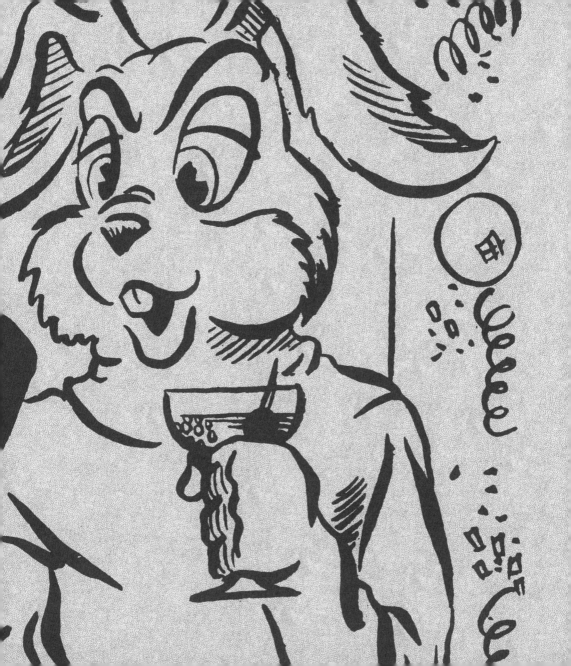

KEEP THE RIVER ON YOUR RIGHT

by Tobias Schneebaum

have been walking around barefoot since the day I got here and calluses instead of cuts are beginning to form. It seemed ridiculous to me to go around naked and have sneakers on my feet.

The thought of nakedness did not occur to me until I saw a young woman making a garment of leaves. She tied a batch of these into a kind of skirt and wrapped it around her waist and thighs. She walked to the river, floated her way across, returned a few minutes later and then dropped the skirt at the water's edge. The carelessness, the inattention with which she discarded the leaves, brought back into my mind the first time I had seen a naked woman. When I was young, thirteen or fourteen, I went, against my father's wishes, to a WPA art school on Union Street in Brooklyn. I had heard of naked models, had seen forbidden photos of them, yet somehow it was never anything that I would see myself, nothing that could become a part of my life. When I sat there in class on that first summer day a young woman came out from behind a screen wrapped in a robe, it seemed impossible that she would stand up on that platform and drop the robe. She took it off, I flushed, blood pounded in my head and I trembled and felt that every eye in the room was turned on me. Casually, I hoped casually, I got up and went to the window and breathed in deeply. Some minutes later, I sat down on my stool, looked straight at the model, picked up my piece of charcoal and began to draw.

It is a strange and surprising way of life here, and I am always learning and seeing new things. About half the women are pregnant. The other day I was out sketching. As I was coming back I saw one of these women alone digging a hole at the edge of a field. She knelt over the hole, her knees wide apart. She let out a groan and a great wet mass dropped down. She sang a long, high-pitched note and another woman came and knelt with her. The mother picked up the baby and they filled in the hole. I followed them to the river, where they washed the child and then took up the body of a small jaguar which had been lying there and allowed the blood from its slit throat to drip down onto the infant's head. They went back to the hut, passing by my three friends with bows and arrows without nodding to them. Later, I saw her working at the fire with the baby asleep in a cradle on her back.

I lay down in my compartment with the other men, thinking of the sketches I had done and watching Michii brush his hair with a densely thistled pod. Darinimbiak began to giggle and slapped Michii on the back and thighs and took up his penis and pulled at it and caressed the testicles. He leaned over and slapped my leg, pulled at the end of my penis and pointed to the woman who had given birth that afternoon and shoved at Michii's back, and hugged him from behind, telling me that Michii had become a father. Michii himself gave no sign of pride or pleasure, and though the mother and child were no more than ten feet away, at the edge of the nearest fire, he made no move toward them. After we had eaten, he got up and went out, passing his child on the way, glancing down for only an instant.

We live apart here, the men and the women. There are children and pregnancies. Yet in the middle of the night no one moves from his partition to seek out a partner. A partner is there next to you, huddled up to you, arms and legs around you. ■

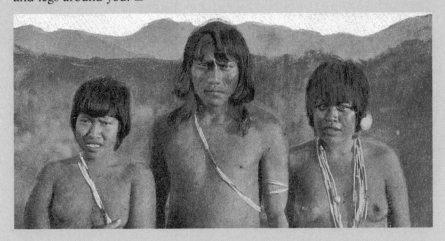

—Written in 1969 about a voyage into the Peruvian jungle in 1955.

Now Dig This

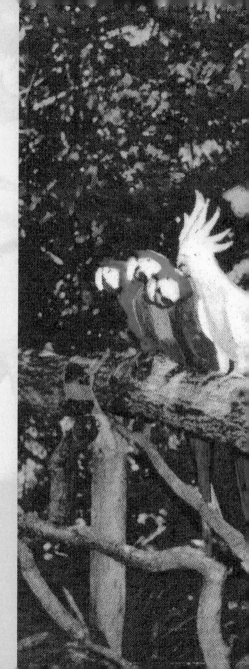

young archaeologist was sent to a remote part of Africa to help with a dig there.

"I'm sure you'll like it here, Digby," a colleague told him on arrival. "On Friday nights we get an enormous amount of booze from the village and have a great time."

"I don't drink," said Digby.

"Oh. Well, I'm sure you'll love Saturdays. We bring in a gang of really *wild* girls from the village and have an orgy."

"I'm not really keen on that sort of thing," said Digby.

His colleague frowned. "I say, you're not *queer*, are you?"

"Of course not," snapped Digby.

"Pity. You won't enjoy Sunday nights, either."

—From *There Was a Young Wench*, (1970) by Seymour Legge.

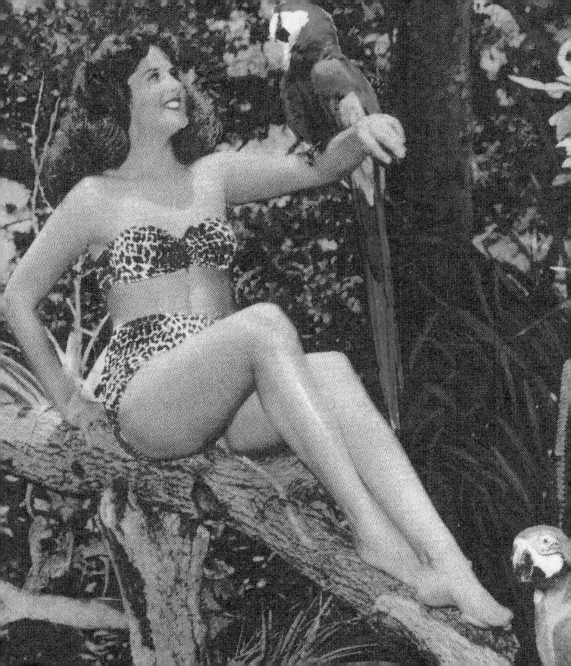

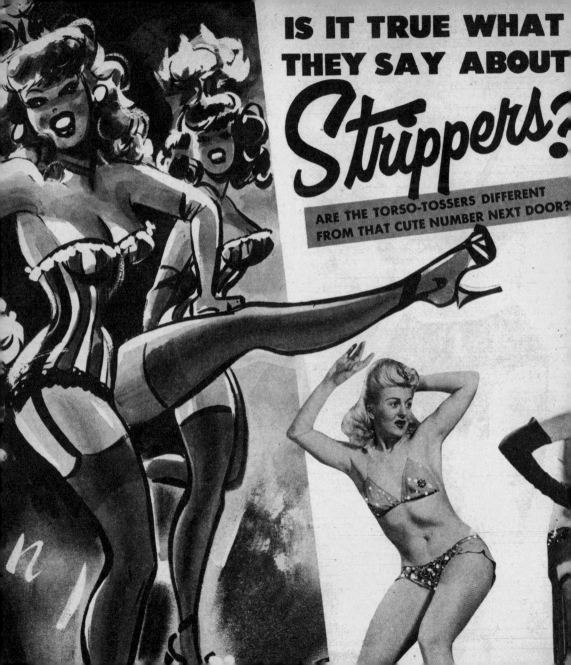

IS IT TRUE WHAT THEY SAY ABOUT *Strippers?*

ARE THE TORSO-TOSSERS DIFFERENT FROM THAT CUTE NUMBER NEXT DOOR?

ARE THE queens of the runway as wiggly offstage as they are when they are doing their stuff onstage or at a honky tonk, or a sizzling night club?

Is it true that none of the leading peelers ever wears a bra? Are they all out to marry a wad of dough? These are only a couple of the questions the boys have about the torso-tossers! Every guy you meet wonders about his favorite stripper. Is she embarrassed when she removes her flimsy costume, while the men whistle and yell?

Well, we interviewed a lot of top hip-flippers, and we came up with some fascinating answers! One cute little bundle of busy curves giggled and said, "I love it when I'm onstage and the boys in the balcony shriek when I take off a bit of this or that! I got nothing to hide, and my chassis is somethin' to be proud of!"

One tall, redheaded torso-tosser had this to say, "Listen, Buster, when I peel I'm workin', same as any steno in an office, but my work stops when the show's over! If some joker thinks he can get fresh just because I'm a peeler, he'll get a black eye, see?"

"A bra? What's that?" queried a dark-haired stripper. "Why should I wear one? I don't need it, do I, Mister?" All the gals interviewed said they wished their favorite guys had a lotta money, but they were *still* their guys, with or without the mazuma! You believe it?

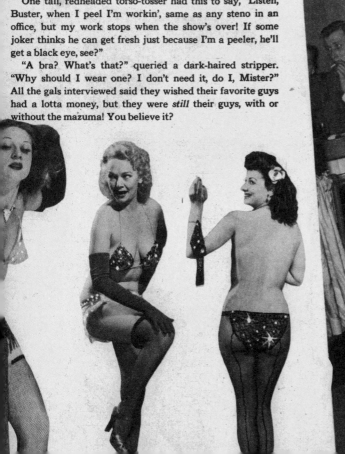

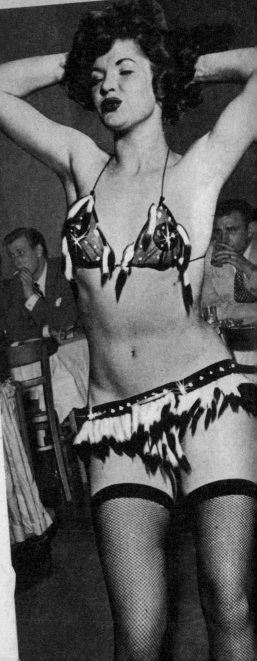

GYPSY

by Gypsy Rose Lee

There was a star on the door, but even so it was the dirtiest dressing room I had ever seen. Greasy make-up towels dragged off the chairs onto the littered floor. Cigarette butts and empty coffee containers and old newspapers were all kicked together with dirty frayed satin shoes under the make-up shelf. Gnats swarmed around a half-empty container of beer, resting on the edge of a filthy sink that was filled with laundry left overnight to soak. Sticky red lip-rouge smudges encircled the entire top of the container. Under each lip-rouge smudge, penciled in with eyebrow pencil, was an initial. The mirrors were broken; their jagged edges reached out like claws. Shreds of net and bits of rhinestones and beads hung by thin strings on nails behind the mirrors.

Mother wrinkled up her nose at the stale, sour odor. "Well," she said, "I guess this will have to do for the time being."

I hesitated in the doorway. "The man told us to take one of the empty rooms," I said.

Mother picked up a make-up towel with two fastidious fingers and dropped it into an overflowing can that served as a wastebasket. "I'm not walking up three flights of stairs in any theatre," she said. "Not with my asthma. And not, I might add, in a theatre like this." She sat on the chair and surveyed the untidy make-up shelf. It was a cluttered mess of powder puffs, empty perfume and liquor bottles, black dirty cosmetic stoves, lipsticks with no tops, coldcream and powder cans with no lids and nasty hairbrushes and combs. One comb, with several teeth missing, had been used to stir a container of coffee and it was still in the container, the cold coffee engulfing it.

The girls and I moved a few of the sweat-stained sleazy costumes to make

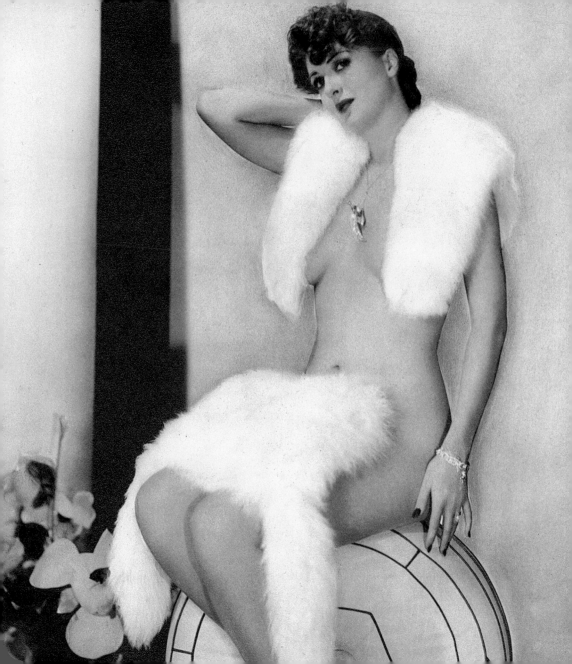

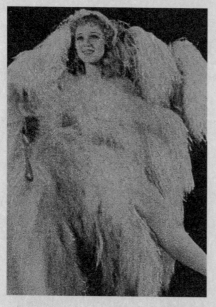

room on the hooks for ours. Nancy lined up the gilded guns beside the wall and I took Porky out of his bag and tied him to a pipe under the sink, along with the dogs.

Ruby held a glittering patch of rhinestones to her thin scrawny neck and gazed at herself in the mirror. "It's kinda big for a necklace," she murmured.

"Put that down!" Mother commanded. "Don't touch anything in this room that doesn't belong to you. You don't know *what* you might catch!"

A blonde woman wearing a black satin dress stood framed in the doorway, her hands on her big, soft-looking hops. "Of all the gawdamned nerve," she said. "The only thing you'll catch around here is a swift kick in the butt if you don't leave my stuff alone!"

Her blond hair stuck out from under a cerise hat; a squirrel coat with the lining torn was flung over her arm. Part of last night's make-up still lingered on her puffy face. She was fatter and older looking than in her picture, but I knew this was Tessie, the tassel twirler.

"Hey, you with the neck," she said to Ruby, "I just paid six bucks for that G string. It's no play toy. Put it down."

Ruby was too frightened to move. The woman strode into the room and snatched the glittering thing from Ruby's hands. "Who told you to come busting in here like it was a public bathhouse?"

"The—door was open," I said. "We've always had the star dressing room and I assumed we'd have—"

"Oh, you did, huh? Well, you can just assume yourselves to hell out.

There's two of us in here already. Now go on—get out—all of ya."

"We'll see who gets out," Mother said. "Girls, unpack the make-up!"

The blonde's anger left her like the air sputtering out of a busted balloon. She flopped onto a chair and let her head hang down between her legs. "Ohmigawd," she moaned, "what a hangover I got. I love my drinks, but they sure don't love me. . . . Why I slop up all that gawddamn beer when I know I got a rehearsal the next day I dunno."

She stirred herself and reached for the container of beer on the sink. Turning it around in her hands until she came to the initial T, she peered in at the dull brownish liquid. "Flat," she announced. "But what the hell, so am I." She held the container to her lips and drank.

Mother picked up the music case. "Stand by for rehearsal," she said; then with a slight curl to her lips, she added, "And no talking to strangers."

The blonde gazed up at her sadly and belched. "I wantta apologize," she said when the belch was over. "I didn't mean to chew your heads off like I did— it's just that I got this lousy hangover— then to find a troupe a acrobats sprawled all over my room—"

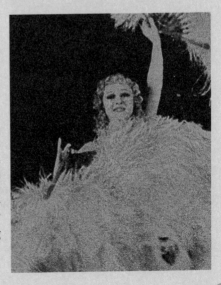

"We aren't acrobats," Mother said witheringly. "We happen to be a vaude-ville act. We were booked into this the-atre by mistake."

"Weren't we all!" the blonde exclaimed; then she belched again.

Mother slammed the door loudly as she left. The girls and I cleared a space on the make-up shelf and laid out our make-up: a can of powder, lip rouge, eye shadow and a can of Crisco. "What's that for?" the blonde asked. "Ya do a little cooking between shows?"

"We use it to take off our make-up," I replied. Mother says it's purer than cold cream."

"Yeah, and a damnsight cheaper," the blonde said. She leaned forward and I made a half-finished gesture to help her. "It's okay, kid, I'm all right." She braced herself with one hand on the make-up shelf and used the other to rummage through a pile of music that was mixed up in the clutter on the floor. With a satisfied grunt, she pulled herself up and stared myopically at the four sheets of music she had salvaged from the pile. She held the music at arm's length, then brought it slowly closer to her face, trying to bring the title into focus. "Does this say 'Digga Digga Doo'?" she asked, shoving the music under my nose. "I can't see a damned thing without my glasses."

It was a lead sheet for "Turn on the Heat." The one she wanted was under it. I lifted it out and gave it to her. She looked at it for a long moment, then she handed it to Dorothy, who was standing closest to the door. "Do me a

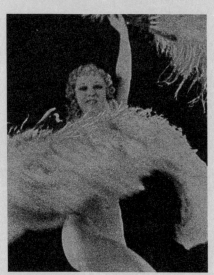

favor, will ya, kid?" she asked as Dorothy's hand closed over the music. "Give this to Benny, the piano player, and tell him to play me a verse and two choruses and to fake anything he wants for the strip—and tell him to ask that chuckle-headed drummer to kindly pick up my bumps—if it ain't asking too much of him."

Dorothy, clutching the music, ran out of the dressing room.

"Gawd, how I hate these damn rehearsals," Tessie said, reaching for the container of flat beer.

A voice called out in the hallway, "Everybody on stage for the opening number. Step on it. We're late gettin' started."

The hallway began filling up with chorus girls wearing red satin brassières and abbreviated pants to match. The pants were open at the sides and held together with pink elastic straps that cut into the flesh, making their hips look corrugated. Long red satin tails were attached to the backs of the pants. The girls' hair was tucked up under red satin skullcaps with tiny horns at the ears. Each girl carried a spear and, as they ran chattering and complaining toward the stage, they poked one another playfully with the pointed ends. One of the girls stopped and began fumbling with the elastic on her pants.

"Hey, Tessie," she said, sticking her head in the doorway. "You got a safety pin? Look at the size a the pants they gamme." She held out the front to show the gap between the pants and her slender body. "Look, I got room in here for a friend."

She had been looking at Tessie; now her eyes traveled over the girls and me. "Who the hell are you?" she asked.

"It's the new vaudeville act," Tessie replied flatly, handing her a safety pin. The chorus girl took a fold in the elastic and stuck the pin through it. "What'll they book next?" she said, fastening the pin. "First it's female wrestlers, then it's Kiki Roberts, and now it's a troupe a silly virgins." She picked up her spear and joined the others in the hallway. Millie ran after her. "We are not!" she yelled.

In a moment the orchestra played the introduction to "Lucky Little Devil" and the chorus girls pranced lackadaisically on stage singing the lyrics of the song in several different keys. The stagehands yelled even louder than the chorus girls as they gave instructions to one another: "Let that tab in a few inches—okay, now tie it off and bring in the front traveler—not so fast—give the broads a chance to finish the number—"

A big fat woman in a gingham dress waddled past carrying a spear. "Dottie," she shouted, "you forgot your spear."

Tessie bounced up from the chair and pushed us away from the door. "Hey, Fudge, wait a minute—I gotta talk to ya about that G string." She hurried over and grabbed up the glittering thing Ruby had been trying on as a necklace. She and the fat woman she called Fudge began examining the patch as though it were the Kohinoor diamond.

"It ain't weighted right," Tessie was saying. "It just don't bump when I do—and it scratches hell outta me."

Fudge held the glittering thing to her broad stomach and did a bump that sent the beads flying wildly. "Works okay for me," she said. "Maybe there's something wrong with your bumper!" She laughed merrily over her little joke but Tessie wasn't amused. "It's no joke to me," she said. "I'm out there bumpin' my brains out and nothing's happening."

Fudge took the G string and waddled out the door. "I'll line the flap with plush," she said.

After she left Tessie turned to us and smiled fondly. "She's a great old girl. Used to be one a the biggest stars in burlesque—but you gotta watch her like a hawk. She'll fob anything off on ya."

A voice screamed off stage, "Kill that damned red flood—I told ya I wanted a bastard pink on them red costumes!"

"Is it always this exciting on opening days?" Nancy bubbled. "I love all the noise and the people running around—"

Tessie didn't answer her. She had spotted Porky, who woke up from his nap in a bad humor. He pulled on his leash and squealed in fury, kicking out with his hoofs at Nancy, who tried to quiet him. "He's hungry," Nancy explained. The dogs began barking, and she raised her voice above the din. "We use him in the act."

"Gawd help us," the blonde said. "And they wonder what happened to vaudeville."

"We're skipping the posing number!" a man yelled in the hallway. "Change into the 'Under the Sea' ballet costumes—'Under the Sea' next!"

Then we heard our music and Mother's voice as she gave the orchestra leader our cues. I tugged at my long, brown stockings and walked down the hallway to the stage. The girls, staying close together, followed me. Two stagehands watched us as we took our places for the opening number of our act. "This is supposed to keep the cops out?" one of them remarked. "Yeah," another one said. "Next week *East Lynne*." ■

—From the 1957 memoir of the self-described "greatest no talent act in the business."

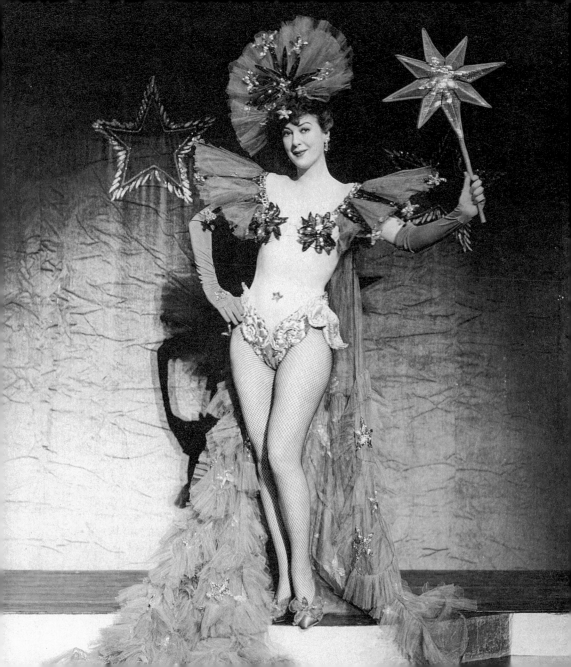

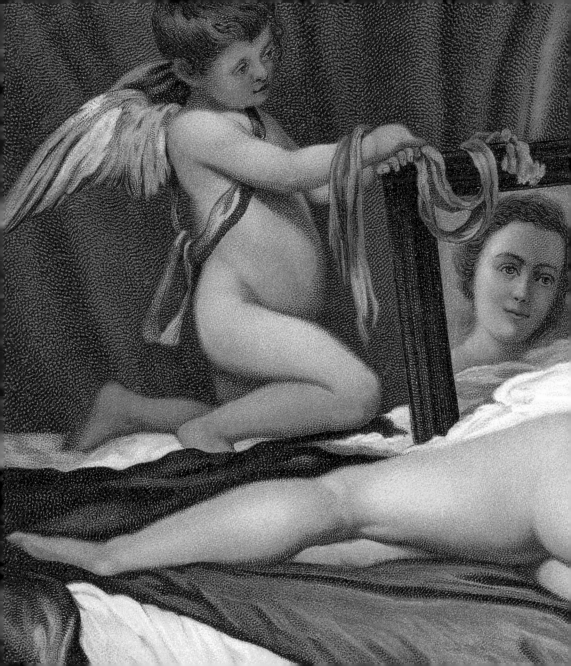

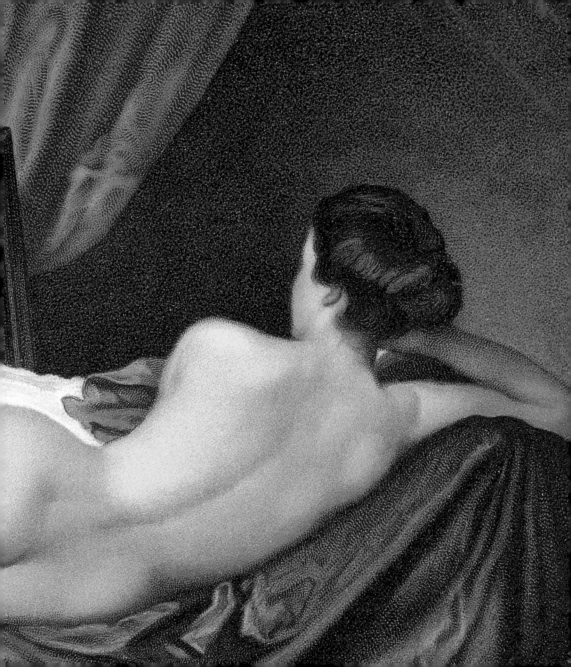

I own a secondhand furniture store and I think my prices are fair,
Course this real cheap guy I know came in one day. Saw this chair he wanted
to buy, but he wouldn't, claimed the price was too high. So I looked straight
in the eye, and this was my reply. . . If I can't sell it, I'm gonna sit down on it.
I ain't gonna give it away. Now darling if you want it, you're gonna have to
buy it. And I mean just what I say. Now how would you like to find this waitin
at home for you every night. Only been used once or twice but it's still nice
and TIGHT! Whoa. . . So if I can't sell it, I'm gonna keep sittin on it. I ain't
gonna give it away. Now you can't find a better pair of legs in town and a
back like this, huh, not for miles around. And that is why if I can't sell it,
I'm going to recline upon it. Why

should I give it away? Because
it's made for comfort, built for
wear and tear. Where else could you
find such an easy chair! Haa. . . Whoa . . .
If I can't sell it, darling I'm gonna sit down
on it. I don't see the need to give it away.

If I Can't Sell It, I'll Sit on It

Andy Razaf, 1920

Because it's lush, plush, slick and sleek. Darling, a high class speech like
this at any price is cheap! So if I can't sell it, I'm gonna sit back down on it.
Why should I give it away? Now look at this nice bottom, ain't it easy on the
eye, guaranteed to support any weight or size! Whoa. . . If I can't sell it, I'm
just gonna keep sittin on it. Don't ask me to give it away. Now, I have really
had my fill of folks always comin around with their hands stuck out, wantin
something, don't want to give up nothing. Now if you want this, put your hand
in your stash and give me some cash. Now if you want something for free, go
to the Salvation Army, don't come runnin to me. Now this is not Saint Paul's
place, this is Ruth's place. Read my lips. NO FREE TRIPS! And you can look at
me and see I have not been starvin' darling. Now I have a few diamonds that
I haven't even taken off to dust lately. Now you are not getting
anything around here for free. Show me the color
of your money. GOODBYE!

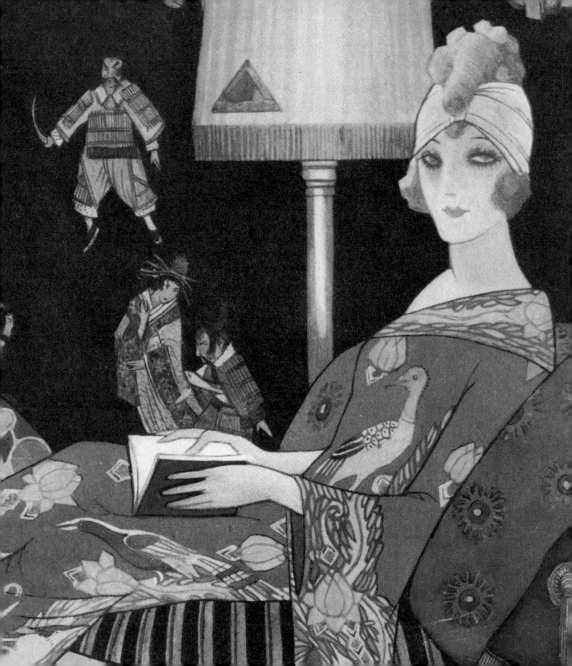

Lawyer Bit.

The burlesque show—a popular early 20th century entertainment—was a mix of ribald routines interspersed with scantily clad women dancing, singing and sometimes stripping. This script belonged to burlesque legend Gypsy Rose Lee.

SETTING: *(Interior of a lawyer's office, two desks, one R. and one L.)*

CAST: *Two comics and Prim.*

(Both Comics enter. Ad. Lib.)

1ST COMIC   Now I know more about law than you do, so let me handle the first case.

2ND   If you handle the first case you will be drunk.

1ST   I handled a case last night and didn't get drunk. *(phone rings)*.

2ND   *(picks up phone)* Start the conversation, this end is ready. What's that? Oh sure, the best lawyers in town.

1ST   That guy admits it.

2ND   Theres a lady coming up and she wants us to handle her case.

1ST   Boy when it comes to handling women's cases, I'm right there.

PRIM   *(enters)* How do you do gentlemen? I'm looking for a smart lawyer.

1ST   Lady, you don't have to look any farther.

PRIM   Oh, but I must have a lawyer with a large diploma.

1ST   Well, you see my partner there ain't got much of a diploma, but I've got one that long. *(measures)*

2ND   What are you talking about, you never saw my diploma.

1ST   Oh yes, I did. I saw you taking a bath last night.

PRIM   You don't seem to understand, I want a diploma that will fit my case.

1ST   Lady, my diploma will fit any woman's case.

2ND   Sit down so we can look into your case.

1ST   No, no, he means, we'll just sit down and tell us about your case.

PRIM   *(sits down)* Well you see gentlemen, I have a large case.

2ND   Well, my partner has a large diploma.

PRIM   Well gentlemen, its like this. My skirt was hanging on the line. (*2nd com. has book and is taking down notes, as evidence*)

1ST   Put the skirt down.

2ND   (*writing in book*) I've got the skirt down.

PRIM   And Mr. Smith's pants were hanging next to my skirt.

1ST   Put the pants down.

2ND   (*writing*) I've got the pants down.

1ST   Now that you have the skirt and pants down, lets get down to business.

PRIM   Mrs. Smith came out of the house and saw my skirt hanging next to Mr. Smith's pants and that made her awful mad.

1ST   Oh hell, yes.

PRIM   Then Mrs. Smith grabbed my skirt and threw it on the ground.

2ND   I got the skirt on the ground.

PRIM   Then Mr. Smith came out of the house and saw that and it made him very mad.

1ST   Oh hell yes, and what did he do?

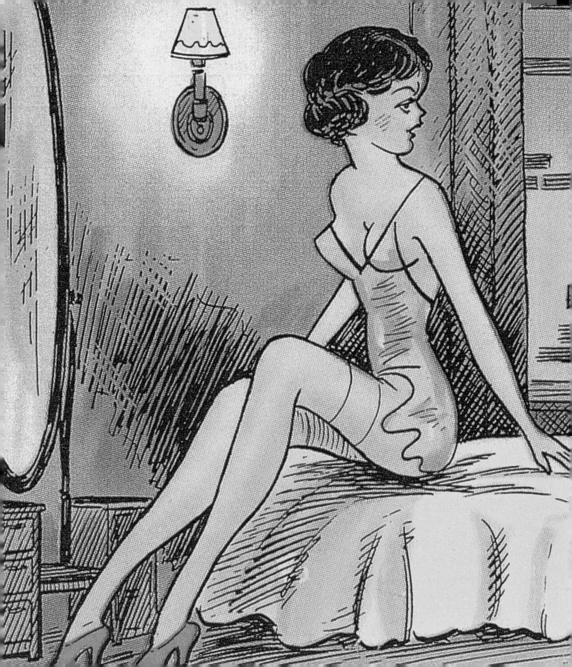

PRIM He suggested only one thing.

1ST What was that?

PRIM He said if I would pick up my skirt he would take down his pants.

2ND He did?

1ST What the hell do you care? Go on and tell us some more.

PRIM Well I picked up my skirt.

2ND And what did Mr. Smith do?

1ST Don't be a damn fool. When a lady picks up her skirt what do you think Mr. Smith would do?

2ND I know.

1ST Well, what did he do?

2ND He took down his pants.

1ST You're not so dumb after all. Now I understand you picked up your skirt and Mr. Smith took down his pants, and then what happened?

PRIM We started to fight, or rather it was more of a wrestle.

1ST Now naturally, when you picked up your skirt and Mr. Smith took down his pants I can see the situation.

2ND I got the situation down.

PRIM And we wrestled and wrestled till we both fell on the ground.

2ND Oh, just a moment, where did you land?

PRIM I landed on the bottom.

1ST Oh hell yes, and Mr. Smith?

PRIM He landed on the top.

1ST Oh naturally, and then what?

PRIM Well, Mr. Smith started to push —

2ND I got the push down.

1ST And what did you do?

PRIM I pushed right back.

1ST Oh yes, and then what happened?

PRIM Well, we both got tired and cleared the matter up.

1ST *(gets up and takes Prim by the hand)*

2ND Hey, what are you going to do?

1ST I'm going to throw my pants in a tree and her skirt on the ground.

2ND And then what?

1ST I'm going to take my pants down, make her pick up her skirt and do the same thing Mr. Smith did. And do a little pushing myself. *(kick exit)*

Black out.

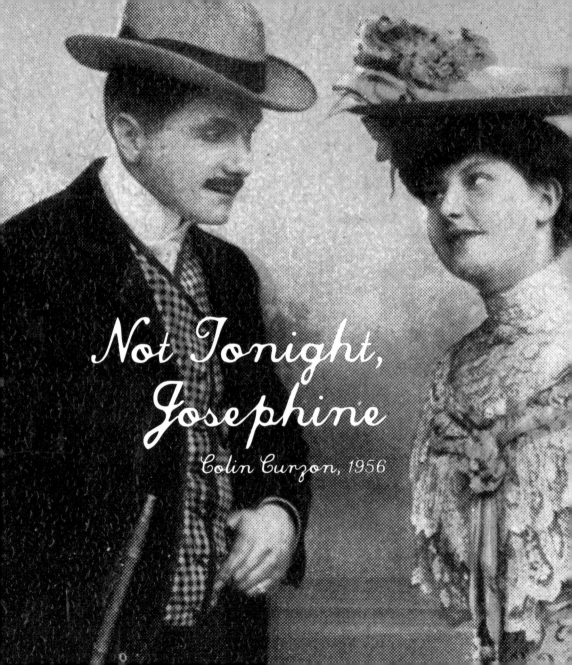

Not Tonight,
Josephine

Colin Curzon, 1956

Though I have an admiration
    for your charming resignation
(There appears no limitation
    to your constant animation)
And a deep appreciation
    of your warm cooperation,
And I find a consolation
    in the pleasing contemplation
Of a coy anticipation
    quite beyond articulation,
Yet forgive the implication
    if I plead disinclination
For the sweet exhilaration
    of a brief amalgamation.
I'll tell you in a phrase, my sweet,
    exactly what I mean:
    . . . Not tonight, Josephine.

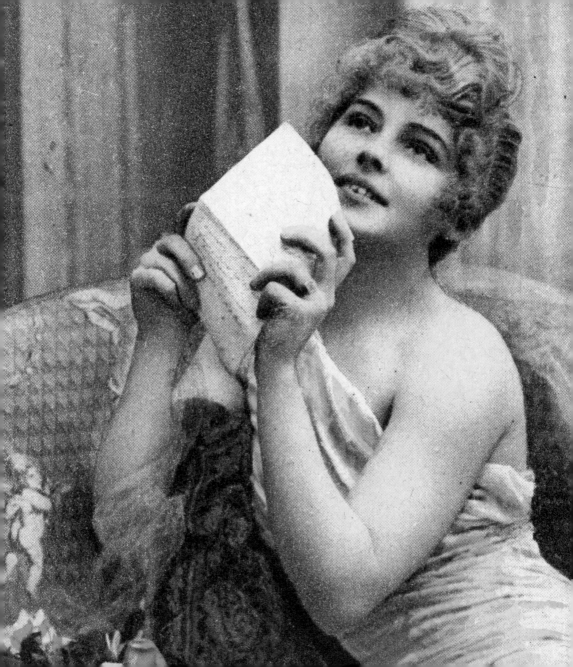

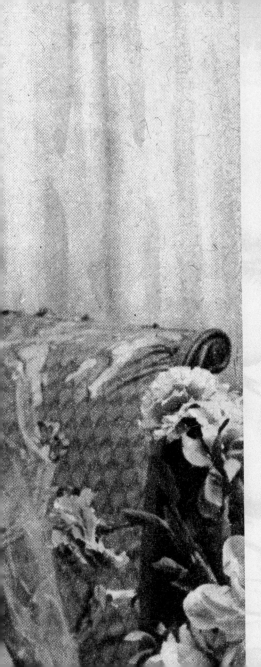

Big Business

Ronald Culver, a somewhat romantic stockbroker, wrote a letter to a pretty client that read:

> Dear Miss Blenkinsop,
> I have a big thing in hand which is expected to rise shortly. If we could get together soon, I'm sure we could make something nice of it."

Eileen Blenkinsop wrote back:

> Dear Mr. Culver,
> Sorry we can't get together at present, as I have my monthly settlement to attend to. But if you can keep your offering standing for a day or two, I can definitely find an opening for it.

—From *There Was a Young Wench*, (1970) by Seymour Legge.

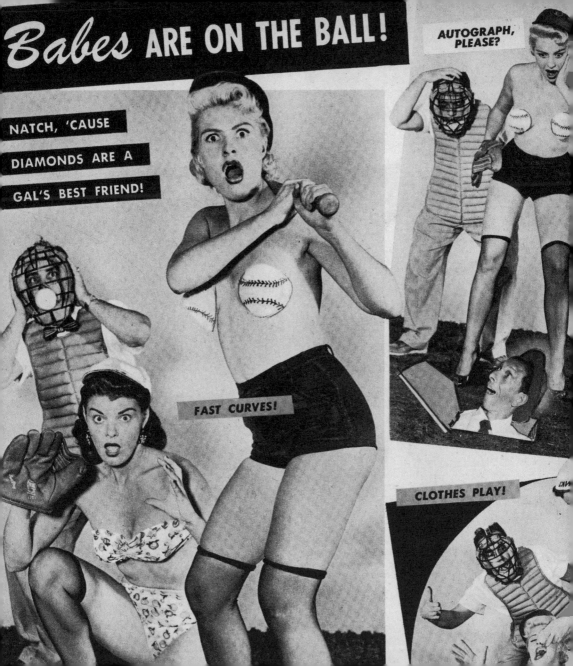

Babes ARE ON THE BALL!

NATCH, 'CAUSE DIAMONDS ARE A GAL'S BEST FRIEND!

AUTOGRAPH, PLEASE?

FAST CURVES!

CLOTHES PLAY!

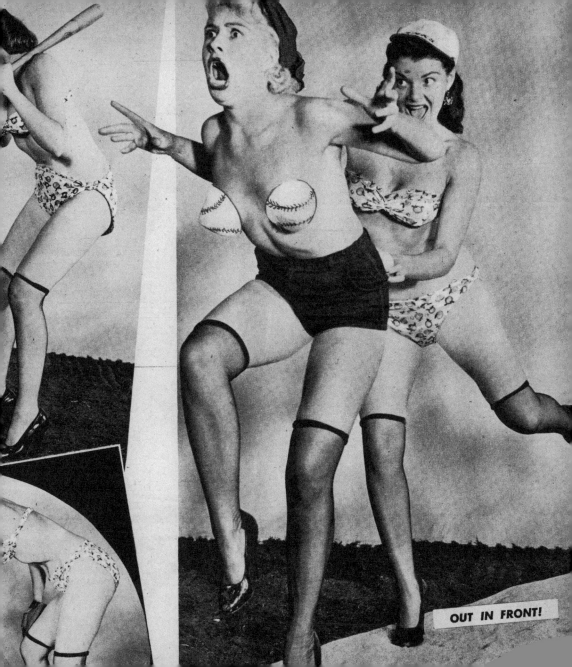

OUT IN FRONT!

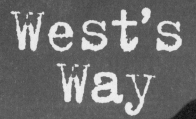

West's Way

Mae: How tall are you?

Man: Six foot seven.

Mae: Well, let's forget about the six foot and talk about the seven inches.

A hard man is good to find.

I only like two kinds of men: domestic and foreign.

I generally avoid temptation unless I can't resist it.

Good sex is like good Bridge. If you don't have a good partner, you'd better have a good hand.

When choosing between two evils I always like to take the one I've never tried before.

Those who are easily shocked, should be shocked more often.

I used to be Snow White but I drifted.

Mae West's first play "Sex,"—the story of an ambitious Montreal prostitute—was on Broadway for over a year when police raided it in 1927, arresting her and the cast. After being convicted of producing a work "calculated to excite in the spectator impure imagination," West spent eight days at Welfare Island Women's Workhouse.

Hollywood Hijinks

A string of lurid and murderous debauchery flowed from Hollywoodland in the early 1920s prompting the formation of the "Hays Code" (see page 194), a set of guidelines created to make Hollywood behave—on screen anyway. Here are some of the naughty tales that kept the public glued to their tabloids at the time.

WILLIAM DESMOND TAYLOR Two shots through the heart of this successful Hollywood director on the night of February 1, 1922 lead to a series of stranger-than-fiction revelations. It was discovered that he was really William Deane-Tanner, a prominent antiques dealer who had suddenly and completely "vanished" from his life in New York (abandoning his socialite wife and daughter) in 1908; his secretary, Edward Sands, had multiple aliases along with a "false" cockney accent; his valet, an illiterate, bisexual black man who had been arrested for indecency involving under aged boys, would, from time to time "introduce" said boys to his employer; he had bedded many of his starlets including 17-year old screen idol Mary Miles Minter

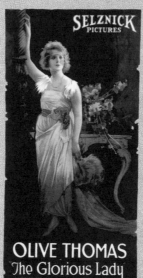

SELZNICK PICTURES

OLIVE THOMAS
The Glorious Lady

and her mother—carrying on those affairs simultaneously, along with at least one other. Newspaper accounts reported that he had been seen at both homosexual hangouts and opium dens. The murder was never solved.

OLIVE THOMAS Winner of 1914's "Most Beautiful Girl in New York City" contest, Ziegfeld Follies showgirl, cover girl, Vargas girl, Broadway and Hollywood star was found dead on the floor of her Paris hotel in September 1920. Gossip had it that after a night of carousing in the infamous Montmartre area while on her honeymoon she drunkenly, and unfortunately, drank a vile of mercury bichloride (prescribed to treat her beloved's chronic syphilis). Another account, however, claimed that she'd been out all night looking for heroin for her husband and apparently partook herself—to deadly consequences.

ROSCOE "FATTY" ARBUCKLE

Perhaps the most popular and well paid actor of his era— garnering a $1 million per year contract from Paramount and rivaled only by Charlie Chaplin— Arbuckle took a fateful break from his hectic schedule Labor Day weekend 1921. An excess of wine, women, fame and money collided at the party he threw at the St. Francis Hotel in San Francisco. Before it was over the young actress Virginia Rappe was being carried out covered in blood. "This is the chance I've waited for for a long time," an eyewitness reported Fatty saying as he led the drunken Rappe into the hotel bedroom. But the encounter with the, some guess, too-well-hung (or maybe just too heavy?) Fatty went terribly wrong and Rappe died three days later of a burst bladder. Rumors ranged from improper use of a champagne bottle to a

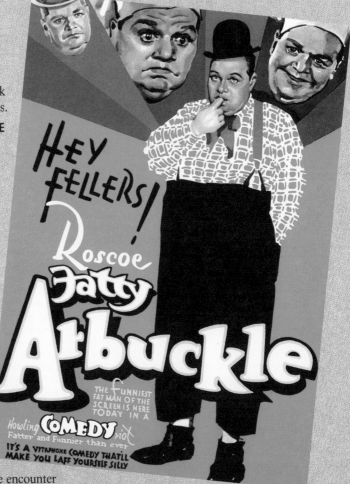

HEY FELLERS!

Roscoe Fatty Arbuckle

THE FUNNIEST FAT MAN OF THE SCREEN IS HERE TODAY IN A

Howling COMEDY Riot
Fatter and Funnier than ever
IT'S A VITAPHOXE COMEDY THAT'LL MAKE YOU LAFF YOURSELF SILLY

botched abortion, and charges of rape and attempted murder were filed. Eventually Arbuckle was acquitted of all charges, but it was too late. His career was ruined.

Hays Code of 1930

The public outcry following a string of Hollywood scandals in the 1920s—a salacious mix of sex, drugs and murder—prompted the formation of what was to become the Motion Picture Association of America. Headed by Will Hays, a former Postmaster General, the Association issued a set of guidelines designed to curb the production of racy and violent films coming out of Hollywood.

One of its main principles was: no picture shall be produced that will lower the moral standards of those who see it.

Here are some specifics:

★ Excessive and lustful kissing, lustful embraces, suggestive postures and gestures, are not to be shown.

★ Passion should so be treated that these scenes do not stimulate the lower and baser element.

★ Seduction or rape . . . are never the proper subject for comedy.

★ Sex perversion or any inference to it is forbidden.

★ Miscegenation (sex relationships between the white and black races) is forbidden.

★ Out of a regard for the sanctity of marriage and the home, the triangle, that is, the love of a third party for one already married, needs careful handling. The treatment should not throw sympathy against marriage as an institution.

★ The treatment of bedrooms must be governed by good taste and delicacy.

★ Impure love must not be presented as attractive and beautiful. It must not be presented in such a way to arouse passion or morbid curiosity on the part of the audience. It must not be made to seem right and permissible. It must not be detailed in method and manner.

★ Dances which suggest or represent sexual actions, whether performed solo or with two or more; dances intended to excite the emotional reaction of an audience; dances with movement of the breasts, excessive body movements while the feet are stationary, violate decency and are wrong.

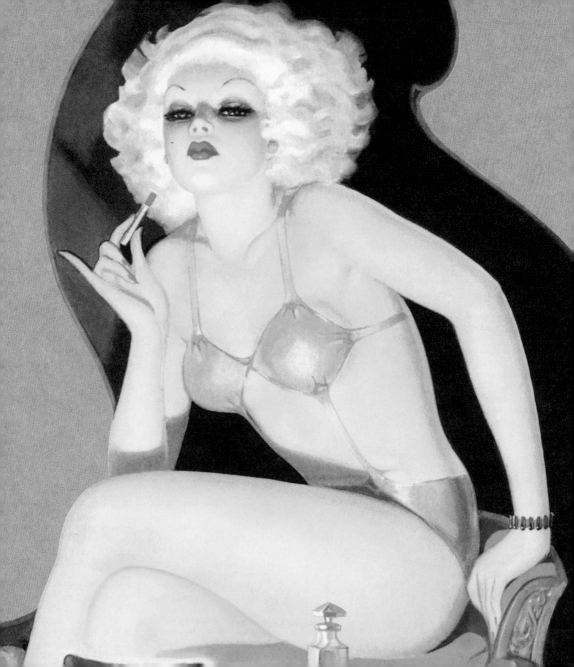

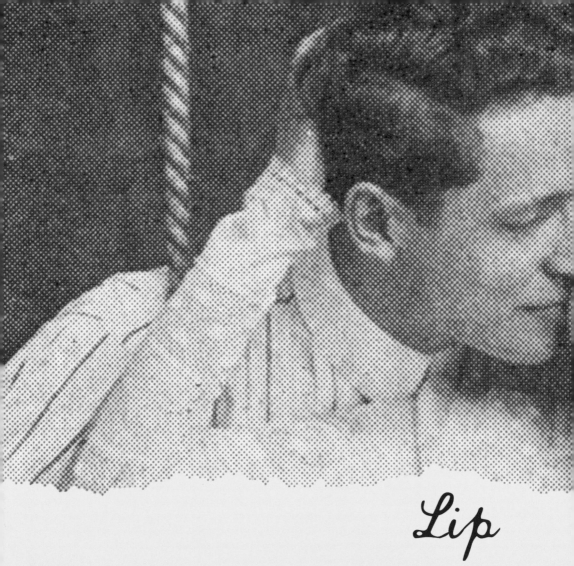

Lip

J. V. Cunningham, c. 1960

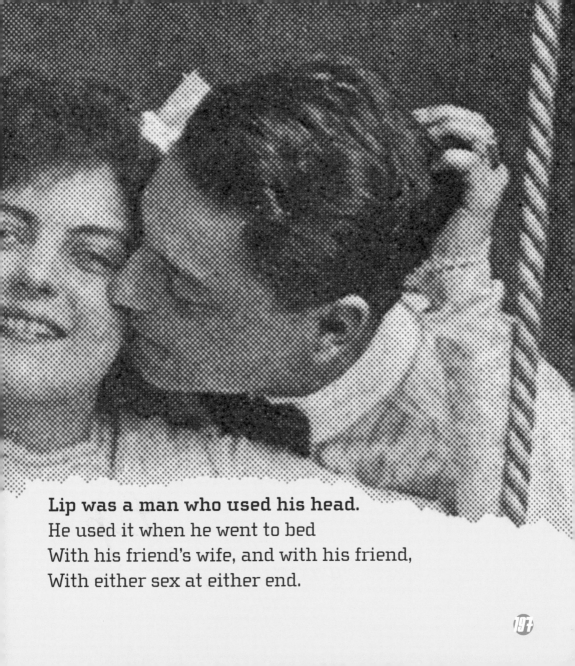

Lip was a man who used his head.
He used it when he went to bed
With his friend's wife, and with his friend,
With either sex at either end.

The Proposition

Paul Blackburn, 1960

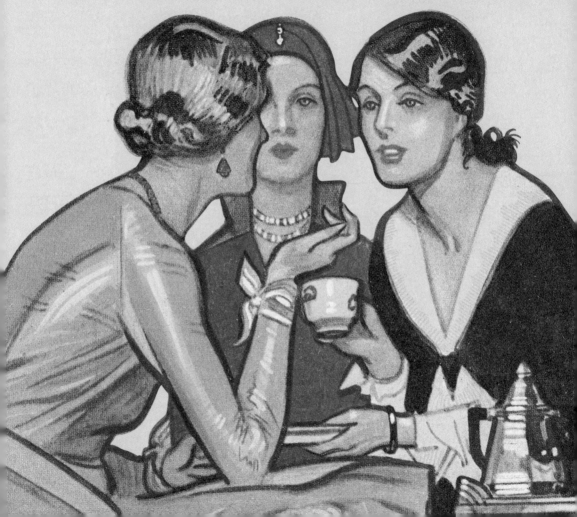

After she

had complained about
men

nearly a solid hour
to her friend's mother
she

was visiting her friend
and her friend's mother
in the country, her

girlfriend left the house
to look for the cat
and she

continued the re-
petitive argument which
her friend's mother

listened to patiently
without comment
until (while)

her daughter was gone
out, (looking for
the cat)

    and she said for the
    100th time how really
    awful bastards

    men were, and didn't she
    (the mother) think there
    WAS

something else to be in-
terested in, or
wasn't it

time to try something
new, the mother
after a long silence

said: "It wouldn't
be new
to me, but I'm

ready anytime you are."
The girlfriend
returning (with the cat)

was a trifle con-
fused when her friend in-
sisted she had to catch the
        late bus home (there

was some editing she
HAD to do). "I hope she wasn't
offended, or anything,"

the mother, after having
driven the girl to her bus
explained

to her daughter, on
the way home the very
probable reason her

friend had left to
go back to the city
so sudden-like

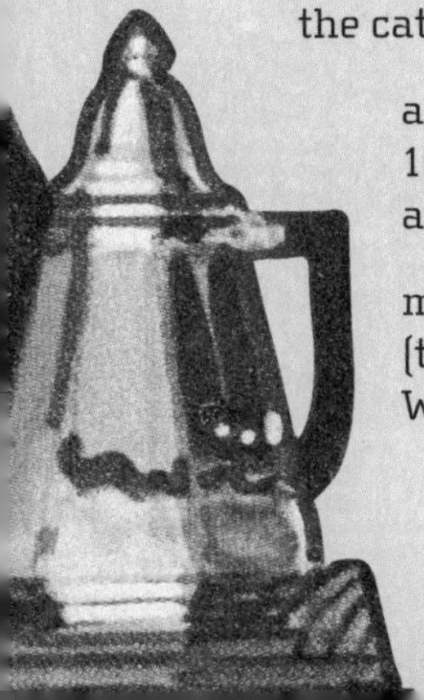

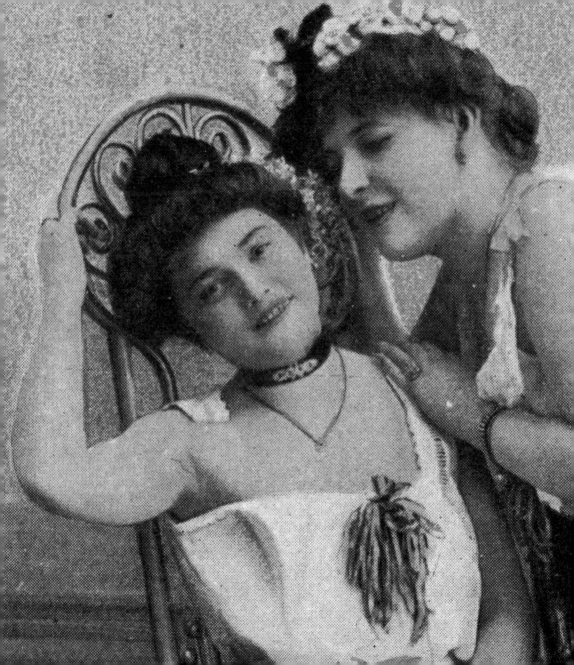

Rumoresque Senum Severiorum

Marcus Argentarius, c. 60 b.c.

It was this way:

I'd been going for weeks with this girl,
Alkippê her name was; well, so
One night I manage to get her up to my room.
That's all right,
Though our hearts are cloppety-clopping like mad
For fear we'll be caught together.

Well,
Everything's fine, you know what I mean, when
All of a sudden the door pops
And in pokes her old mother's sheep-head:
"Remember, daughter," she bleats, "you and I go halves!"

A MASTERPIECE OF EROTICA FROM THE UNCENSORED TEXT OF "LADY CHATTERLEY'S LOVER"

The electrifying text of D. H. Lawrence now comes alive in the powerful and passionate narration of this great record. Constance Chatterley bares her most intimate emotions as she tells of her erotic raptures and sexual fulfillment. We witness a miraculous transformation. At one time frustrated and dissatisfied with the sterility of her life, Lady Chatterley is drawn to Mellors, the gamekeeper. Yet she is fearful, vulnerable in her longing desire.

"I put my arms round him under his shirt, but I was afraid. Afraid of his thin, smooth naked body, that seemed so powerful, afraid of the violent muscles. I shrank, afraid. And when he said something with a sort of a little sigh: something in me quivered, my spirit stiffened in resistance: stiffened from the terribly physical intimacy, from the peculiar haste of his possession.

"And I felt him like a flame of desire, yet tender, and I felt myself melting in that flame. I let myself go. I felt him against me with silent, amazing force and assertion, and I let myself go to him. I yielded with a quiver that was like death, I went all open to him. And oh, if he were not tender to me now—how cruel. For I was all open to him and helpless!"

Gradually she surrenders to a complete and overwhelming sexual freedom. Exulting in every sensual delight, she describes her relationship in great detail.

"I lay quite still, in a sort of sleep, in a sort of dream. Then I quivered as I felt his hand groping softly, yet with queer thwarted clumsiness among my clothing. Yet the hand knew, too, how to unclothe me where it wanted. He drew down the thin silk sheath, slowly, carefully, right down and over my feet. Then with a quiver of exquisite pleasure he touched the warm soft body . . ."

Lady Chatterley's words are vividly dramatized by the sultry-voiced "Ilona," an actress of great talent and beauty. She kindles the flame of this stirring text, breathing life into a characterization of Lady Chatterley that will long be remembered as a masterpiece of dramatic interpretation.

A most beautiful and brilliant musical score provides a lush background for this record.

"Lud of Hollywood," one of the foremost exponents of the pastel medium in the fine arts field, was commissioned by Fax to produce the cover of this record album.

—From the liner notes, 1962, Fax Records.

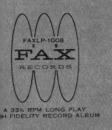

EROTICA SERIES #4

$4.98

FAXLP-100B

FAX
RECORDS

A 33⅓ RPM LONG PLAY
HI FIDELITY RECORD ALBUM

The Erotic Delights Of Lady C.

*A masterpiece of erotica from the
uncensored text of
"Lady Chatterley's Lover"*

Sex Crimes of the Pilgrims

by Brian Alexander

The Pilgrims have a reputation as a pretty dour bunch, and, true to their reputation—according to a remarkable online archive of texts and scholarly commentaries assembled by anthropologists at the University of Virginia—they spent a lot of time thinking about how to punish lust.

Though there was no formal criminal code at the time of the first Thanksgiving in the autumn of 1621, everybody knew what was expected because they were intimate with the source of Pilgrim law, the Bible. (Many old sex laws still on the books are, in fact, taken almost straight out of the Bible.) Passages from Leviticus provided Pilgrims with some sex laws, and prescribed punishments. Poor Thomas Graunger, a teenage farm boy, perhaps flush with the surge of hormones, turned to those he knew best. Governor William Bradford recounted the tale: "He was this year detected of buggery, and indicted for the same, with a mare, a cow, two goats, five sheep, two calves and a turkey . . ." Thomas was executed as dictated by Leviticus.

Punishments for sex crimes were brutal, but records show that threat of suffering did not deter all passionate puritans.

"Mary, the wife of Robert Mendame, of Duxborrow" was put on trial for "dalliance diverse times with Tinsin, an Indian . . ." And "Edward Holman hath been observed to frequent the house of Thomas Sherive at unreasonable times of the night . . . which is feared to be of ill consequence . . . the Court has therefore ordered . . . Edward Holman . . . henceforth do no more frequent or come at the house of the said Sherive, nor that the wife of the said Sherive do frequent the house or company of the said Holman, as either of them will answer it at their perils."

The court had no idea why Holman was going to visit Sherive or his wife (or both? Hmm . . .) but those who create sex bans often have the best imaginations.

It wasn't all severity at Plymouth. The Courts did attempt fair trials and some accused were found innocent. Sometimes punishments were skipped out of mercy.

Perhaps such mercy was a nod to human nature. After all, according to some estimates, up to 50 percent of Plymouth colonists had premarital sex, despite the laws. Some were gay or bisexual. There were bad marriages, cheating wives, teenagers flooded with hormones. Life was complicated. Does that sound familiar?

—From an article first published on msnbc.com, November 2006.

Here Comes Santa . . .

Because ancient winter solstice rituals—many being celebrations of rebirth and fertility—were incorporated into the Christmas holiday, some current traditions have origins that are a little sexier than you may think.

■ Mistletoe was believed to resemble the genitalia of a Druid god—the white berries (and their gooey content) representing drops of semen.

■ The red berries of the holly tree, also sacred to the Druids, were thought to represent menstrual blood.

■ Evergreen trees were the embodiment of eternal life, fertility and potency to pre-Christian Germanic people . . . and so were seen as big fat green phallic symbols.

■ Ancient Scandinavians celebrated *Jol* (pronounced yule) to honor the god of intoxicating drink and ecstasy—sort of like modern-day office parties. Some sources say that their large, imposing yule log represented the original red-hot poker.

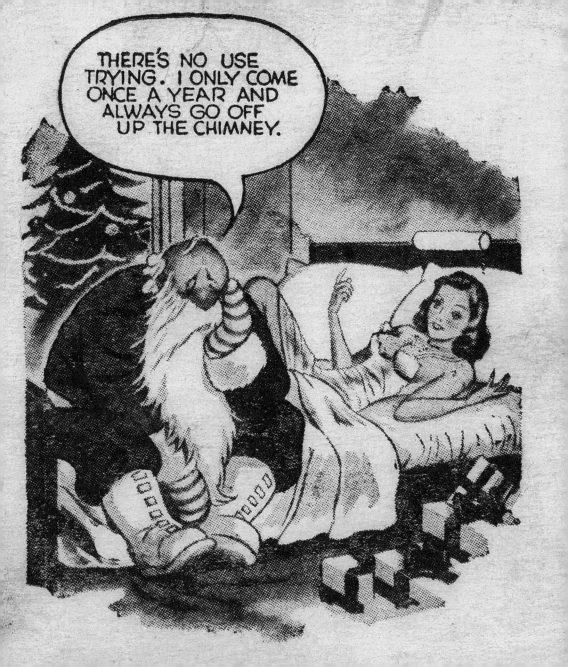

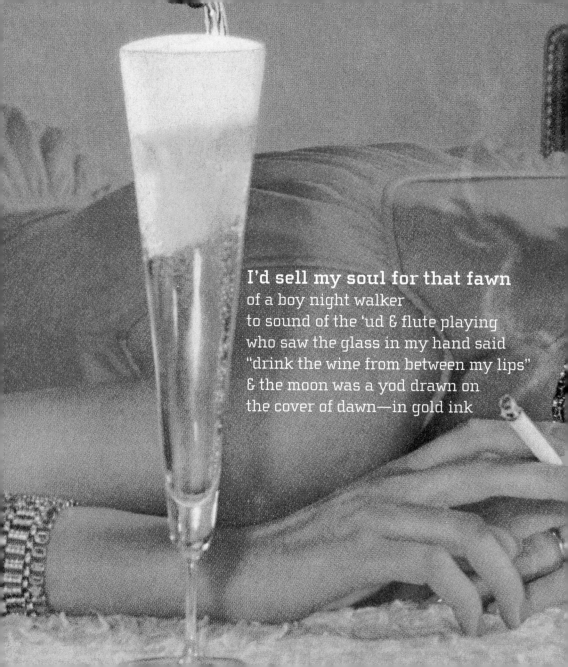

I'd sell my soul for that fawn
of a boy night walker
to sound of the 'ud & flute playing
who saw the glass in my hand said
"drink the wine from between my lips"
& the moon was a yod drawn on
the cover of dawn—in gold ink

Love Poem

Samuel ha' Nagid, c. 1000

THE LUSTFUL TURK

by Anonymous

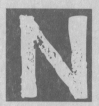o sooner were the Captain and Eliza withdrawn than the Dey rose from the couch, walking leisurely towards me, and laid hold of my hand which trembled in his grasp. After considering a few moments, he chucked me under the chin, and said in good English, that Mohamet had been kind in blessing him with so fair a slave as myself. I was not much surprised to hear the Dey speak English, the Captain having spoken it so well, but the terror his address gave me cannot be described, and indeed good reason I had for my apprehensions. Directly he had spoken, he was leading me towards the couch, but I instantaneously drew back, on which without further ceremony he caught me round the waist, and spite of the resistance I made, forced me to it; then seating himself he drew me to him, and forced me to seat myself upon his knees. If it had been in my power to have resisted, the excess of my confusion alone would have prevented my throwing any effectual obstacle in the way of his proceedings. Directly he had got me thus he threw one of his arms round my neck, and drew my lips to his, closing my mouth with his audacious kisses. Whilst his lips were as it were glued to mine, he forced his tongue into my mouth in a manner which created a sensation it is quite impossible to describe. It was the first liberty of the kind I ever sustained. You may guess the shock it at first gave me, but you will scarcely credit it when I own that my indignation was not of long continuance. Nature, too powerful nature, had become alarmed and assisted his lascivious proceedings, conveying his kisses, brutal as they were, to the inmost recesses of my heart. On a sudden new and wild sensations blended with my shame and rage, which exerted themselves but faintly; in fact, Silvia, in a few short moments his kisses and his tongue threw my senses into a complete tumult; an unknown fire rushed through every part

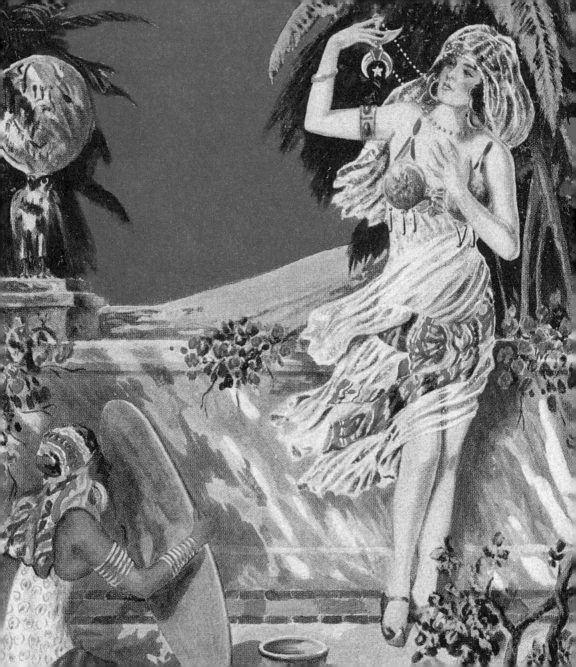

of me, hurried on by a strange pleasure; all my loud cries dwindled into gentle sighs, and spite of my inward rage and grief, I could not resist. So wanting strength for self-defense, I could only bewail my situation. I told you he had me on his knees, with one of his arms round my neck—finding how little I resisted, and having me thus with our lips joined, his other hand he suddenly thrust under my petticoats. Aroused by this vital insult, I strove to break from his arms, but it was of no use, he held me firm, my cries and reproaches he heeded not! If by my struggles I contrived to free my lips, they were quickly regained again; thus with his hand and lips he kept me in the greatest disorder, whilst in proportion as it increased I felt my fury and strength diminish; at last a dizzy sensation seized on every sense. I felt his hand rapidly divide my thighs, and quickly one of his fingers penetrated that place which God knows, no male hand had ever before touched. If anything was wanting to complete my confusion, it was the thrilling sensation I felt, caused by the touches of his finger. What a dreadful moment was this for my virtue! With all the highest notions of the charms of that dear innocence which I was doomed to be so soon deprived of, dreading how strange then it was that pleasure should overcome with such fear about me. Why did this not instantly snatch me from the pleasure? I wished some help would come to save me from the danger, but had no sooner formed the wish, than a kiss, and his finger created a contrary emotion, and each following kiss grew more and more pleasing, till at last I almost wished nothing might oppose my absolute defeat. In blushing at what I felt, I blush to write, I longed to feel more. Without an idea what I panted for could be, I eagerly awaited the instruction until the impetuous ardor began to be too powerful for the senses.

Finding that I made no attempt to withdraw my lips from his thrilling pleasure, his arm which was around my neck he removed to my waist. Being thus drawn by it more strongly to his bosom, his right arm became closely confined between his body and mine, my hand being placed and held firmly between his thighs. Whilst in this position, I felt something beneath his clothes gradually enlarging and moving against my hand; from the length I felt against my arm, I judged it to be very long and thick also. If I had wished to remove my hand from its position I could not; and so wonderful was the fascination I felt from the mere touch of this unknown object, I think I could not have removed my hand had it been perfectly at liberty. Without knowing what it was, every throb created in me a tremor unaccountable. I little dreamed the dreadful anguish I was doomed to experience by that which my hand was warming and raising to life.

By this time the Dey had satisfied himself of my being a virgin. Sunk as I was in every soft idea, still I had not been able to silence the unfortunate monitor within my breast, who though hitherto unsuccessful was yet reproaching me for my weakness. The Dey fully perceiving the impression he had made, resolved to take immediate advantage of it. But how shall I describe what I still blush to think of—but it must be done—he withdrew his hand from between my thighs, forced me on my back on the couch, and in an instant turned up my clothes above my navel. Thus all my secret

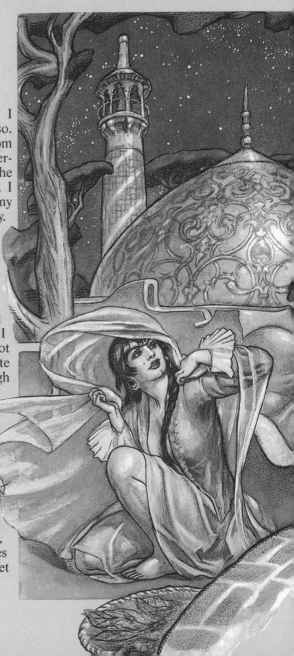

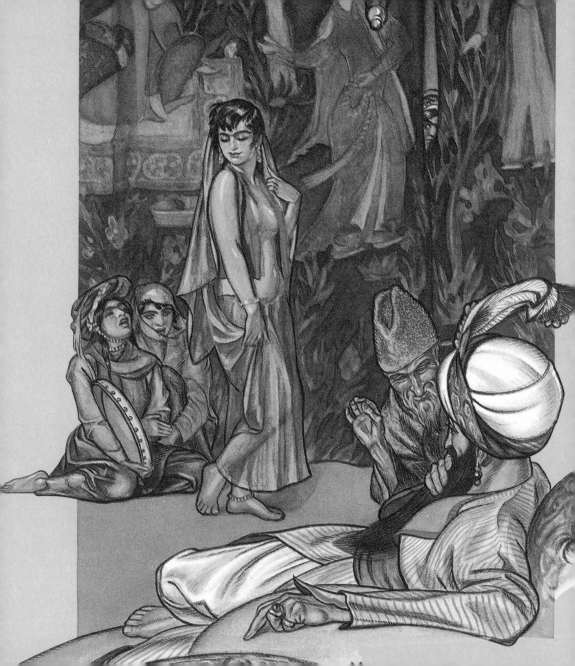

charms became exposed to his view. Exhausted as I was and lost in desire, I could make no further resistance; his hands quickly divided my thighs and he got between them. During my struggles my neckerchief had become loose and disordered; he now entirely removed it, leaving my neck and breast quite bare.

Although I could scarcely keep my eyes open from the tumult of my senses, still I could not help observing as he was on his knees between my thighs that he was divesting himself of his lower garments before he laid on me. For the first time in my life I caught a view of that terrible instrument, that fatal foe to virginity. With unutterable sensations I felt his naked glowing body join mine, again my lips were glued to his, softening me to ruin with his inflamed suctions. In a delirium little short of pleasure, panting with desire I waited my coming fate. I really think if at this moment he had committed my seduction, I should not have regretted my loss of virtue—but no, it was decreed on being deprived of my innocence I should be entirely free of all those soft desires he had so powerfully excited, and that I should suffer during my defloration every anguish a maid can feel, personal as well as mental. But to my unfortunate tale. The Dey had properly fixed himself to do that which I ought but most certainly at the moment did not dread. No, not even as I felt his daring hand fixing the head of his terrible instrument where his lascivious fingers had so potently assisted in reducing me to my then passive state, I own I felt it even with pleasure stiffly distending my, until that moment, untouched modesty. But on the very instant when I had willingly resigned everything to what I then considered my fixed destiny, his eyes, whose lustre and expression I could scarcely sustain the sight of, on a sudden were filled with languor. He seemed as it were abashed, and kissing me with less violence, he grew by degrees even weaker than myself: suddenly I felt my thighs overflowed by something warm that spurted in torrents from his instrument, and at last he sunk in my arms in a kind of trance. ■

—First published in 1828.

215

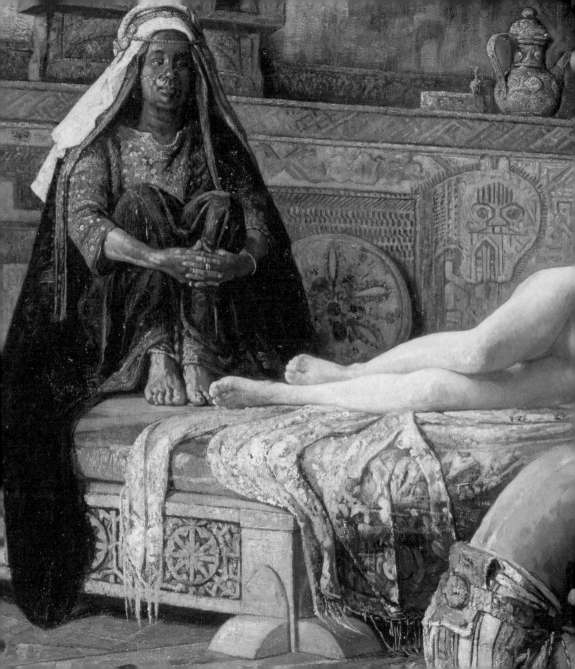

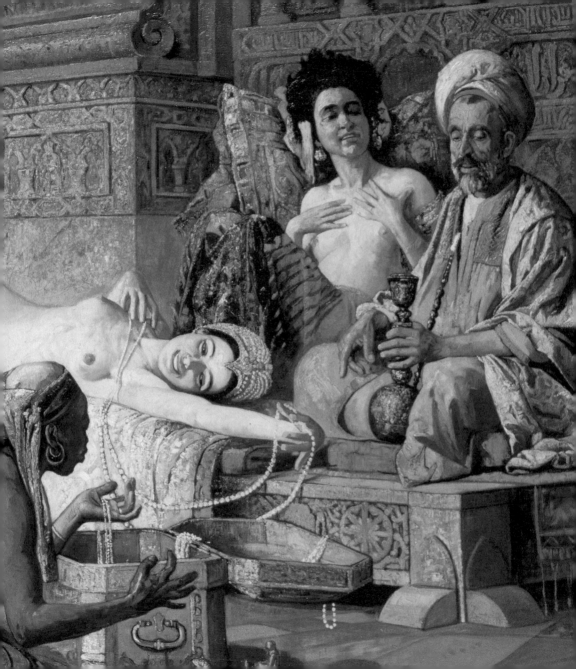

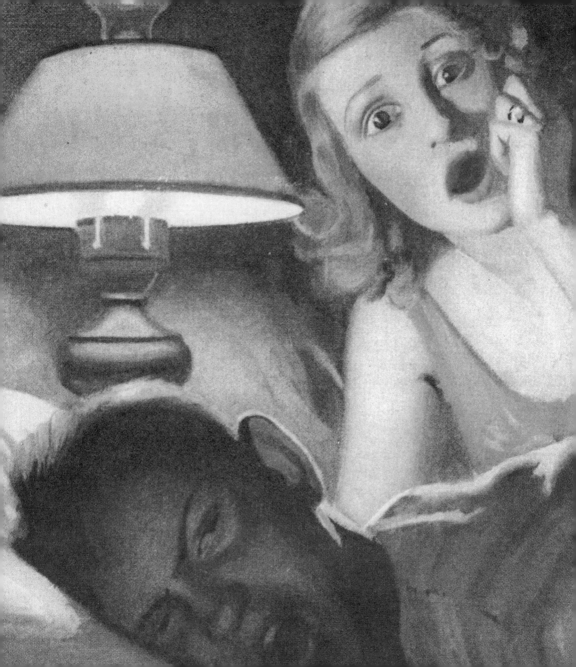

The Rummy Cove's Delight

c. 1833

Ye wives when you marry, of course you expect
That your husbands with something in front will be deck'd;
And should he be gifted with what's rather small,
It's better than if he had nothing at all.
But the story I tell you is true, 'pon my life,
It's found out a woman has married a wife,
Who was strong, who was hearty, was stout and was tall,
But to please her poor spouse she had—Nothing at all.

She liv'd as a groom, and the housemaid she wed,
And the very first night that they went into bed,
The wife she did turn round her face to the wall,
For she knew that her husband had—No—thing at all.
Then they laid all the night, and no doubt they both sigh'd,
For a good strapping drayman their charms to divide;
'Twas very provoking it so did befall,
That one for the other had—Nothing at all.

In a dockyard this husband did work for some years,
Undiscover'd to be a female, it appears;
And but for an accident, there is no doubt,
This secret of secrets had ne'er been found out
But it happen'd one day, that this female did die,
And the searchers were sent for, who quickly did spy,
That instead of a three-square gimblet or awl,
She'd a-a what-do'ye-call-it,—a nothing at all.

A GLAMOUR GIRL
IN BRIEF ATTIRE...

CAN SET
A FELLOW'S
THOUGHTS
AFIRE!

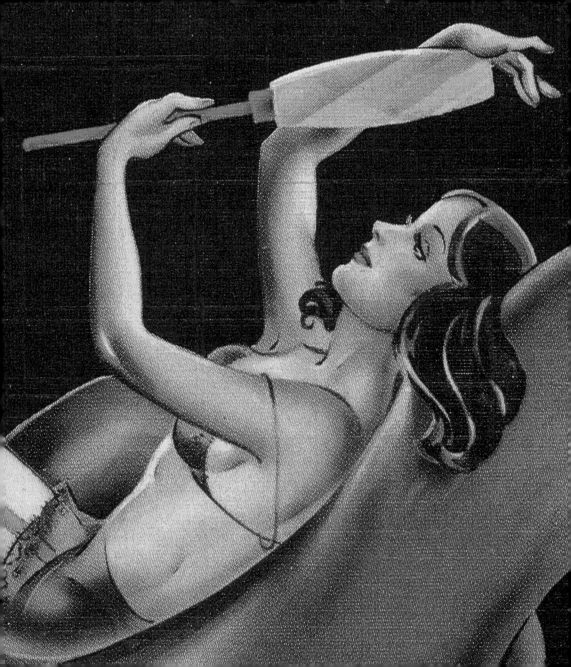

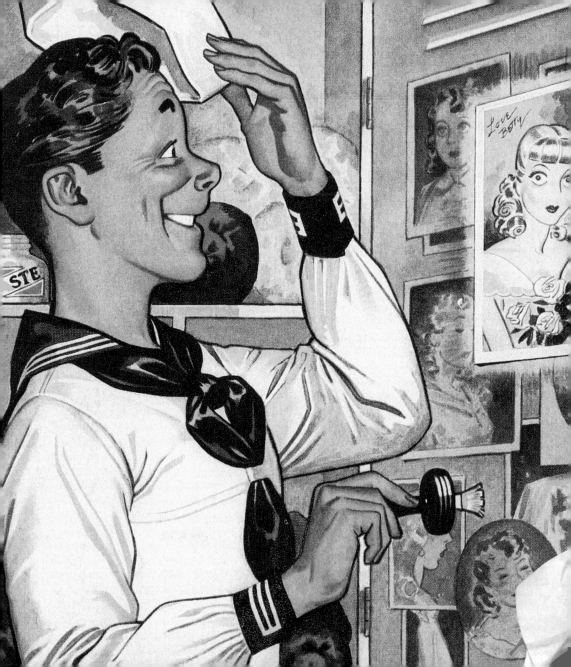

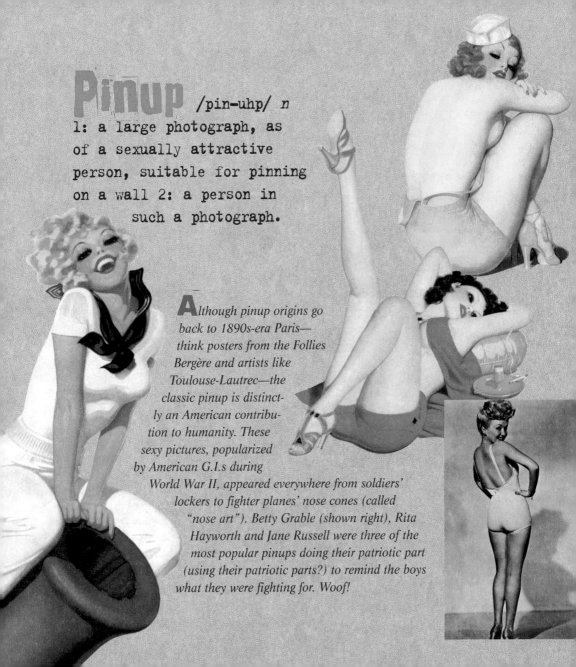

Pinup

/pin-uhp/ *n*

1: a large photograph, as of a sexually attractive person, suitable for pinning on a wall 2: a person in such a photograph.

Although pinup origins go back to 1890s-era Paris— think posters from the Follies Bergère and artists like Toulouse-Lautrec—the classic pinup is distinct- ly an American contribu- tion to humanity. These sexy pictures, popularized by American G.I.s during World War II, appeared everywhere from soldiers' lockers to fighter planes' nose cones (called "nose art"). Betty Grable (shown right), Rita Hayworth and Jane Russell were three of the most popular pinups doing their patriotic part (using their patriotic parts?) to remind the boys what they were fighting for. Woof!

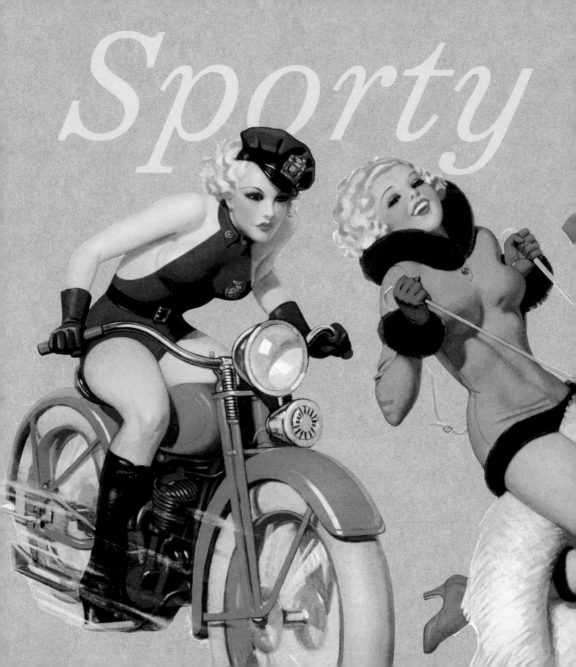

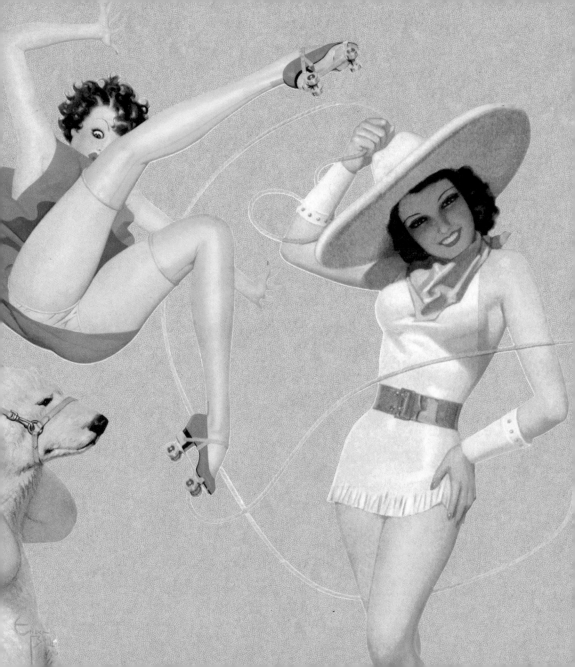

EN LA NOCHE

by Ray Bradbury

ll night Mrs. Navarrez moaned, and these moans filled the tenement like a light turned on in every room so no one could sleep. All night she gnashed her white pillow and wrung her thin hands and cried, "My Joe!" The tenement people, at 3 A.M., finally discouraged that she would *never* shut her painted red mouth, arose, feeling warm and gritty, and dressed to take the trolley downtown to an all-night movie. There Roy Rogers chased bad men through veils of stale smoke and spoke dialogue above the soft snorings in the dark night theater.

By dawn Mrs. Navarrez was still sobbing and screaming.

During the day it was not so bad. Then the massed choir of babies crying here or there in the house added the saving grace of what was almost a harmony. There was also the chugging thunder of the washing machines on the tenement porch, and chenille-robed women standing on the flooded, soggy boards of the porch, talking their Mexican gossip rapidly. But now and again, above the shrill talk, the washing, the babies, one could hear Mrs. Navarrez like a radio tuned high. "My Joe, oh, my poor Joe!" she screamed.

Now, at twilight, the men arrived with the sweat of their work under their arms. Lolling in cool bathtubs all through the cooking tenement, they cursed and held their hands to their ears.

"Is she *still* at it!" they raged helplessly. One man even kicked her door. "Shut *up*, woman!" But this only made Mrs. Navarrez shriek louder. "Oh, ah! Joe, Joe!"

"Tonight we eat out!" said the men to their wives. All through the house, kitchen utensils were shelved and doors locked as men hurried their perfumed wives down the halls by their pale elbows.

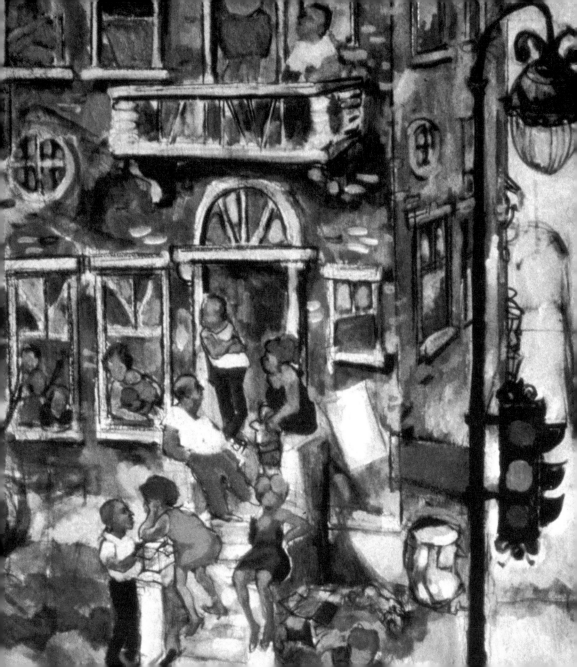

Mr. Villanazul, unlocking his ancient, flaking door at midnight, closed his brown eyes and stood for a moment, swaying. His wife Tina stood beside him with their three sons and two daughters, one in arms.

"Oh God," whispered Mr. Villanazul. "Sweet Jesus, come down off the cross and silence that woman." They entered their dim little room and looked at the blue candlelight flickering under a lonely crucifix. Mr. Villanazul shook his head philosophically. "He is still on the cross."

They lay in their beds like burning barbecues, the summer night basting them with their own liquors. The house flamed with that ill women's cry.

"I am stifled!" Mr. Villanazul fled through the tenement, downstairs to the front porch with his wife, leaving the children, who had the great and miraculous talent of sleeping through all things.

Dim figures occupied the front porch, a dozen quiet men crouched with cigarettes fuming and glowing in their brown fingers, women in chenille wrappers taking what there was of the summer-night wind. They moved like dream figures, like clothes dummies worked stiffly on wires and rollers. Their eyes were puffed and their tongues thick.

"Let us go to her room and strangle her," said one of the men.

"No, that would not be right," said a woman. "Let us throw her from the window."

Everyone laughed tiredly.

Mr. Villanazul stood blinking bewilderedly at all the people. His wife moved sluggishly beside him.

"You would think Joe was the only man in the world to join the Army," someone said irritably. "Mrs. Navarrez, *pah!* This Joe-husband of hers will peel potatoes; the safest man in the infantry!"

"Something *must* be done." Mr. Villanazul had spoken. He was startled at the hard firmness of his own voice. Everyone glanced at him.

"We can't go on another night," Mr. Villanazul continued bluntly.

"The more we pound her door, the more she cries," explained Mr. Gomez.

"The priest came this afternoon," said Mrs. Gutierrez. "We sent for him in desperation. But Mrs. Navarrez would not even let him in the door, no matter how he pleaded. The priest went away. We had Officer Gilvie yell at her, too, but do you think she listened?"

"We must try some other way, then," mused Mr. Villanazul. "Someone must be—sympathetic —with her."

"What other way is there?" asked Mr. Gomez.

"If only," figured Mr. Villanazul after a moment's thought, "if only there was a *single* man among us."

He dropped that like a cold stone into a deep well. He let the splash occur and the ripples move gently out.

Everybody sighed.

It was like a little summer-night wind arisen. The men straightened up a bit; the women quickened.

"But," replied Mr. Gomez, sinking back, "we are all married. There is no single man."

"Oh," said everyone, and settled down into the hot, empty river bed of night, smoke rising, silent.

"Then," Mr. Villanazul shot back, lifting his shoulders, tightening his mouth, "it must be one of *us!*"

Again the night wind blew, stirring the people in awe.

"This is no time for selfishness!" declared Villanazul. "One of us must *do* this thing! That, or roast in hell another night!"

Now the people on the porch separated away from him, blinking. "*You* will do it, of course, Mr. Villanazul?" they wished to know.

He stiffened. The cigarette almost fell from his fingers. "Oh, but I—" he objected.

"You," they said. "Yes?"

He waved his hands feverishly. "I have a wife and five children, one in arms!"

"But none of us are single, and it is your idea and you must have the courage of your convictions, Mr. Villanazul!" everyone said.

He was very frightened and silent. He glanced with startled flashes of his eyes at his wife.

She stood wearily weaving on the night air, trying to see him.

"I'm so tired," she grieved.

"Tina," he said.

"I will die if I do not sleep," she said.

"Oh, but Tina!" he said.

"I will die and there will be many flowers and I will be buried if I do not get some rest," she murmured.

"She looks very bad," said everyone.

Mr. Villanazul hesitated only a moment longer. He touched his wife's slack hot fingers. He touched her hot cheek with his lips.

Without a word he walked from the porch.

They could hear his feet climbing the unlit stairs of the house, up and around to the third floor where Mrs. Navarrez wailed and screamed.

They waited on the porch.

The men lit new cigarettes and flicked away the matches, talking like the wind, the women wandering around among them, all of them coming and talking to Mrs. Villanazul, who stood, lines under her tired eyes, leaning against the porch rail.

"Now," whispered one of the men quietly, "Mr. Villanazul is at the top of the house!"

Everybody quieted.

"Now," hissed the man in a stage whisper, "Mr. Villanazul taps at her door! Tap, tap."

Everyone listened, holding his breath.

Far away there was a gentle tapping sound.

"Now, Mrs. Navarrez, at this intrusion, breaks out anew with crying!"

At the top of the house came a scream.

"Now," the man imagined, crouched, his hand delicately weaving on the air, "Mr. Villanazul pleads and pleads, softly, quietly, to the locked door."

The people on the porch lifted their chins tentatively, trying to see through three flights of wood and plaster to the third floor, waiting.

The screaming faded.

"Now, Mr. Villanazul talks quickly, he pleads, he whispers, he promises," cried the man softly.

The screaming settled to a sobbing, the sobbing to a moan, and finally all died away into breathing and the pounding of hearts and listening.

After about two minutes of standing, sweating, waiting, everyone on the porch heard the door far away upstairs rattle its lock, open, and, a second later, with a whisper, close.

The house was silent.

Silence lived in every room like a light turned off. Silence flowed like a cool wine in the tunnel halls. Silence came through the open casements like a cool breath from the cellar. They all stood breathing the coolness of it.

"Ah," they sighed.

Men flicked away cigarettes and moved on tiptoe into the silent tenement. Women followed. Soon the porch was empty. They drifted in cool halls of quietness.

Mrs. Villanazul, in a drugged stupor, unlocked her door.

"We must give Mr. Villanazul a banquet," a voice whispered.

"Light a candle for him tomorrow."

The doors shut.

In her fresh bed Mrs. Villanazul lay. He is a thoughtful man, she dreamed, eyes closed. For such things, I love him.

The silence was like a cool hand, stroking her to sleep. ∎

—This short story, also known as *Torrid Sacrifice*, was written in 1952.

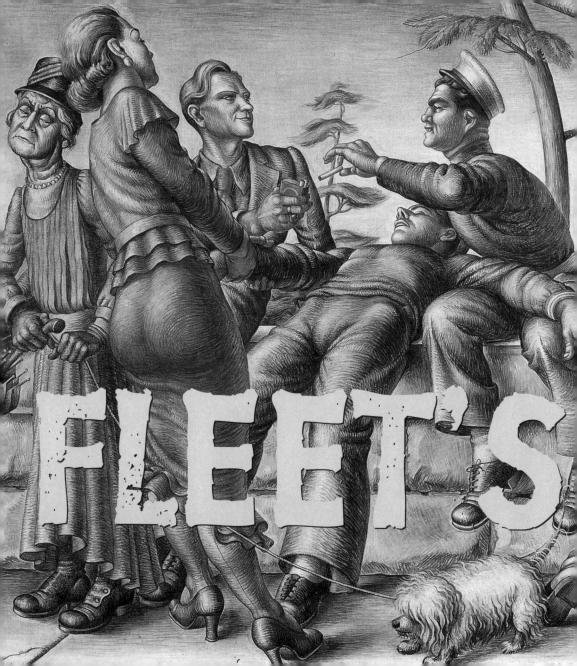

FLEET'S

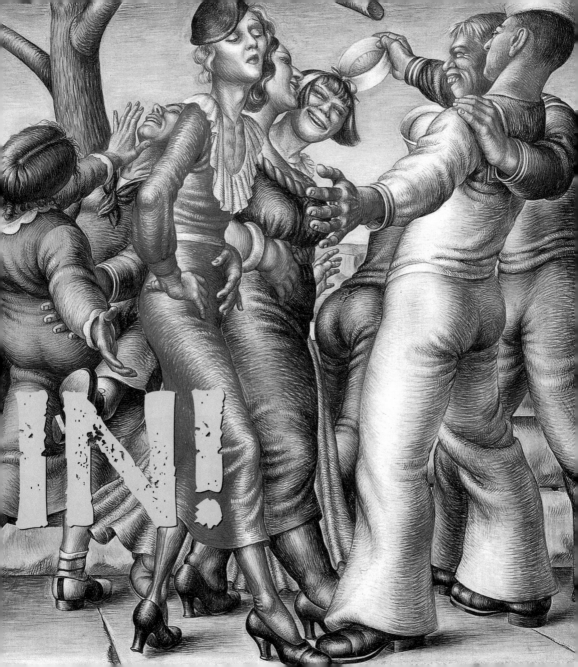

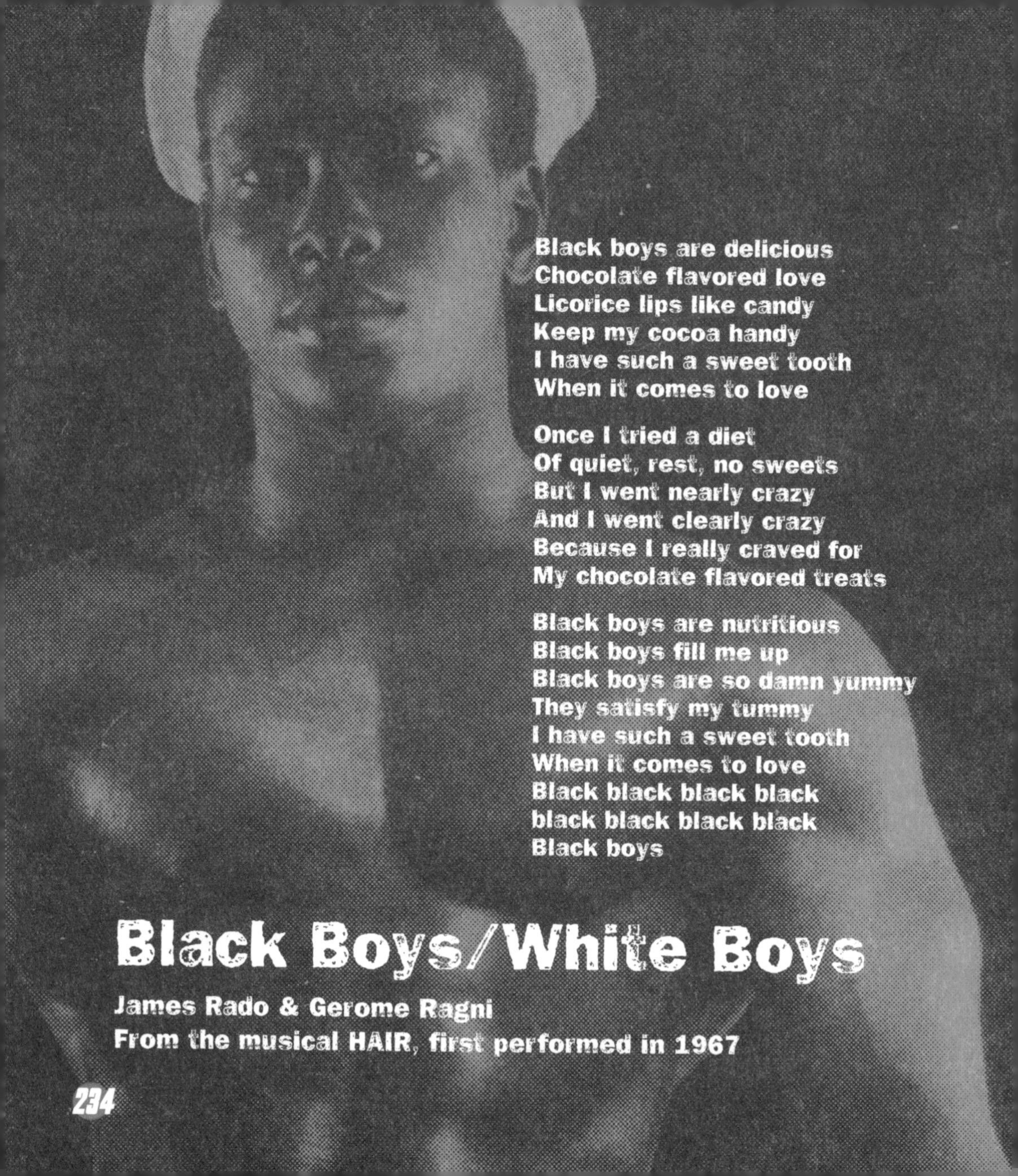

Black boys are delicious
Chocolate flavored love
Licorice lips like candy
Keep my cocoa handy
I have such a sweet tooth
When it comes to love

Once I tried a diet
Of quiet, rest, no sweets
But I went nearly crazy
And I went clearly crazy
Because I really craved for
My chocolate flavored treats

Black boys are nutritious
Black boys fill me up
Black boys are so damn yummy
They satisfy my tummy
I have such a sweet tooth
When it comes to love
Black black black black
black black black black
Black boys

Black Boys/White Boys

James Rado & Gerome Ragni
From the musical HAIR, first performed in 1967

White boys are so pretty
Skin as smooth as milk
White boys are so pretty
Hair like Chinese silk

White boys give me goose bumps
White boys give me chills
When they touch my shoulder
That's the touch that kills

Well, my momma calls 'em lilies
I call 'em Piccadillies
My daddy warns me stay away
I say come on out and play

White boys are so groovy
White boys are so tough
Every time that they're near me
I just can't get enough

White boys are so pretty
White boys are so sweet
White boys drive me crazy
Drive me indiscreet

White boys are so sexy
Legs so long and lean
Love those sprayed-on trousers
Love the love machine

My brother calls 'em rubble
That's my kind of trouble
My daddy warns me "no no no"
But I say "White boys go go go"

White boys are so lovely
Beautiful as girls
I love to run my fingers
And toes through all their curls

Give me a tall
A lean
A sexy
A sweet
A pretty
A juicy
White boy

Black boys!
White boys!
Black boys!
White boys!

Mixed media!

Beefcake

n. Informal 1: Images, especially photographs, of minimally attired men with muscular physiques. 2: Attractive men with muscular physiques, such as those in these images. Origin: 1945–50; beef + cake, modeled on cheesecake.

A hunk of beefcake images were printed from the 1930s to the 1960s in magazines as a sort of above-ground underground way for gay men to bypass antiquated censorship laws and take a peek at some very-nearly-naked brawn. The magazines pretended innocence by presenting wholesome Adonises either promoting fitness and health or enacting classical, "artistic" scenarios. Some of the more popular publications featuring the hubba-hubba he-men were: *Young Physique, Tomorrow's Man, Beach Adonis, Demi-Gods, Muscle Boy, Teen Torso* and *Muscles a Go-Go*. Grrrrrr!

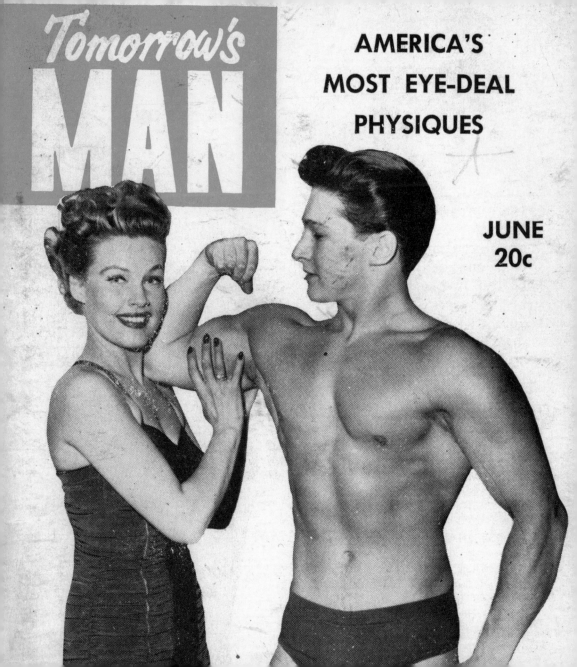

Tomorrow's MAN

AMERICA'S
MOST EYE-DEAL
PHYSIQUES

JUNE
20c

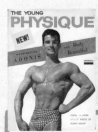
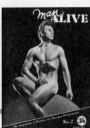
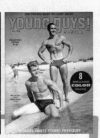

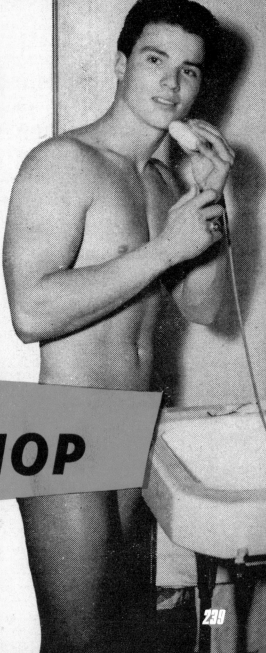

He's not so tall (5′9″) but he's certainly dark and handsome. His name is Glen Bishop and don't be too surprised if you see his name in lights over the door of your neighborhood theater a few years from now.

We'd Like You To Meet
GLEN BISHOP

CLOSE SHAVE: Glen's a stickler for personal hygiene and cleanliness which accounts for his un-flecked skin, glistening hair, and polished teeth. He's not modest at the dinner table either . . .

SODOM OR
THE QUINTESSENCE OF DEBAUCHERY

attributed to John Wilmot, Earl of Rochester

Enter PRICKET *and* SWIVIA *embracing him*

SWIVIA: Twelve months must pass ere you can yet arrive
    To be a perfect man, that is to swive,
    As Pockenello doth
    Your age to fifteen does but yet incline.

PRICKET: You know I could have stript my Prick at nine. *(He shows.)*

SWIVIA: By h—en's a neat one, now we are alone
    I'll shut the door and you shall see my thing. *(She shows.)*

PRICKET: Strange how it looks, me thinks it smells of ling
    It has a beard too, and the mouth's all raw.
    The strangest Creature that I ever saw:
    Are these the Beards that keep men in such aw?

SWIVIA: 't Was such as these Philosophers have taught
    That all mankind into the world have brought.
    't Was such a thing the King our Sire bestir'd
    out of whose whomb we came,

PRICKET: The devil we did.

SWIVIA: This is the ware house of the world's chief Trade,
    On this soft anvil all mankind was made.
    Come 't is a harmless thing, draw near and try
    You will desire no other Death to dye.

PRICKET: Is 't death then?

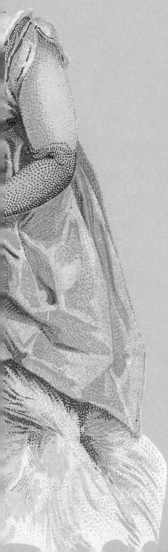

SWIVIA: Ay, but with such plaisant pain,
   That it will tickle you to live again.

PRICKET: I feel my spirits in an agony.

SWIVIA: These are the symptoms of young Letchery
   Does not your Prick stand, and your Pulse beat fast?
   Don't you desire some unknown bliss to taste?

PRICKET: My heart invites me to some new desire,
   My blood boils over.

SWIVIA: I can allay the fire.
   Come little Rogue and on my belly lie *(Lies on her.)*
   A little lower, yet, now, dearest, try.

PRICKET: I am a stranger to these unknown parts
   And never vers'd in Loves obliging arts:
   Pray, guide me, I was ne'er this way before.

SWIVIA: There, can't you enter? Now you've found the door.

PRICKET: Now I am in, and 't is as soft as wool.

SWIVIA: Then move it up and down, you little fool.

PRICKET: I do, o he—ens, I am at my wits' end.

SWIVIA: It 't not such pleasure as I did commend?

PRICKET: Yes. I find Cunt a most obliging friend
   Speak to me sister ere my soul depart.

SWIVIA: I cannot speak, you've stabb'd me to the heart.

PRICKET: I faint, I can't one moment more survive,
   I am dead

SWIVIA: Oh, Brother, but . . . Alive
   And why should you lie dead, to increase my pain,
   Kiss me, dear rogue, and thou shalt live again.

—From the satire first published in the seventeenth century and often
described as "the most obscene play ever written."

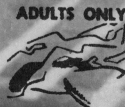

STA

STO

FOR

ME

ADULTS ONLY

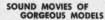
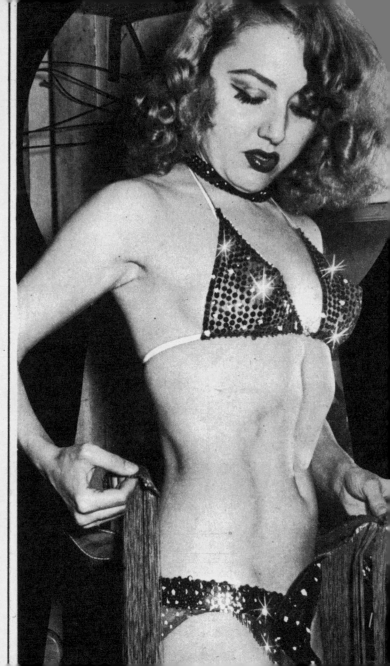

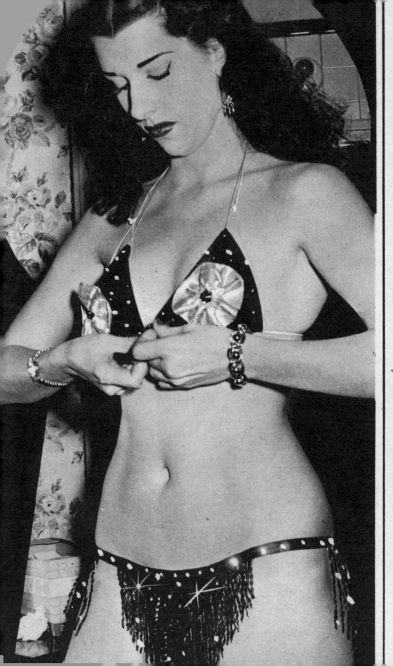

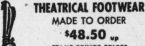
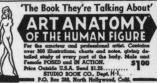

A is for Anatomical Correctness

(part three)

boff, boink, bone, bonk, bop, drill, cream, shag, plow, plug, poke *mount* nail, hammer, ball, pork, schtupp, screw, scrog, play hide the hot dog, dance the horizontal tango, dance the matrimonial polka, dance the mattress jig, fix her plumbing, get busy, get it on, get creamy, get Jack in the orchard *get jiggy with it* have a bit of sugar stick, have a hot roll with cream, have a squeeze and a squirt, have a turn on your back, make whoopee *thread the needle* hide the pickle, mix the baby juice, hide the salami, hide the sausage, feed the kitty, eat the cream puff in the enchanted forest *give the dog a bone* exchange bodily fluids, ride the skin bus in to Tuna Town, trade a bit of hard for a bit of soft, exchange DNA, burp the worm in the mole hole, put the bee in the hive, put the candle in the pumpkin *put a snake on her plane* put sour cream in the burrito, shake the sheets, put Percy in the playpen, shuck the oyster, sink it in, enact God's plan, get your oil changed, get your rocks off, get your chimney swept out *a bit of the old in & out* organ grinding, makin' bacon, mingle limbs, Adam and Eve it, horizontal hula (hustle, mambo, polka, or tango), hot beef injection, beef in yo taco, have a bit of giblet pie, butter the muffin, buzz the Brillo, phallicize someone *plant a man* toss off a batch of baby batter, play doctor, play pickle-me-tickle-me, get a leg over, carnal gymnastics . . .

P is for _____

246

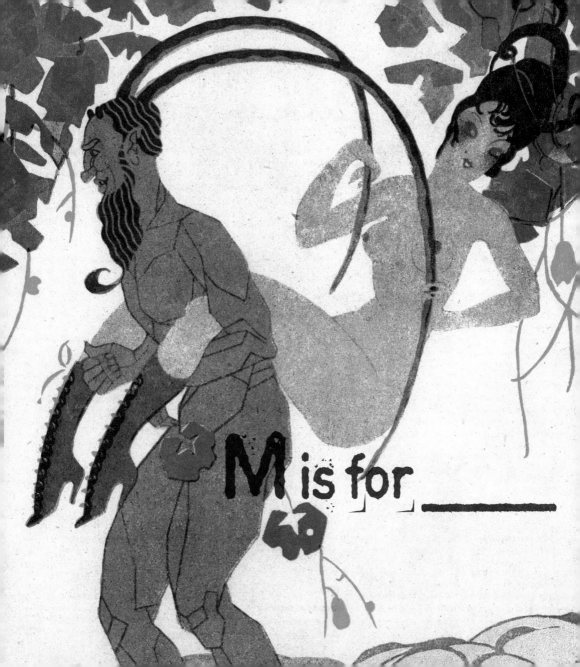

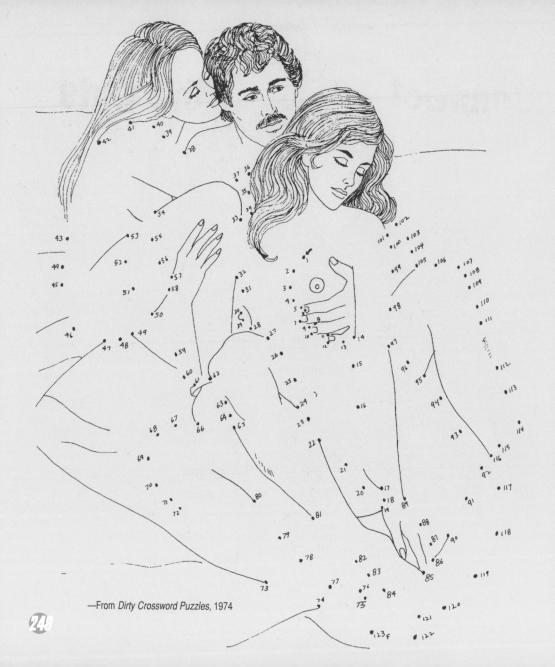

—From *Dirty Crossword Puzzles*, 1974

Connect the Dots

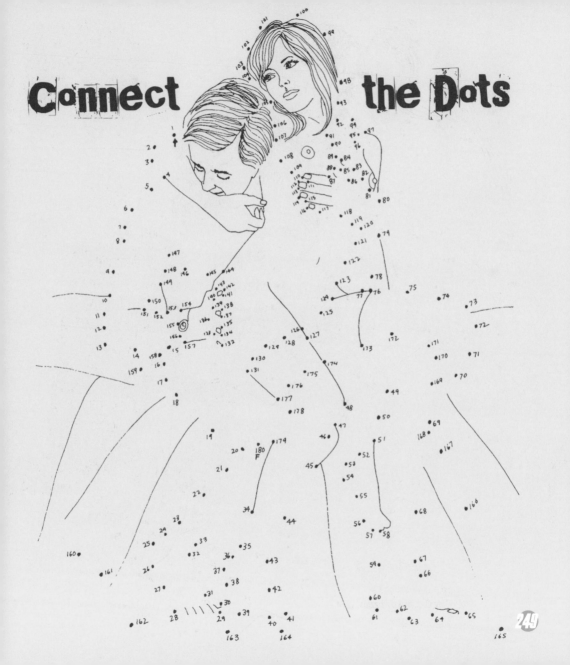

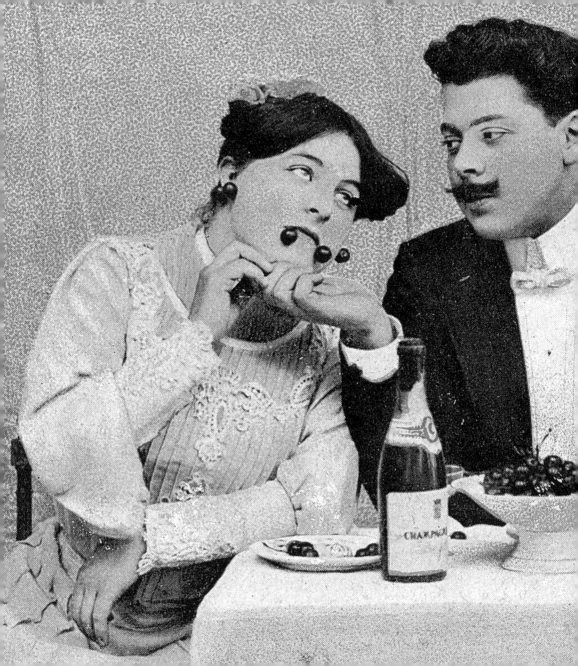

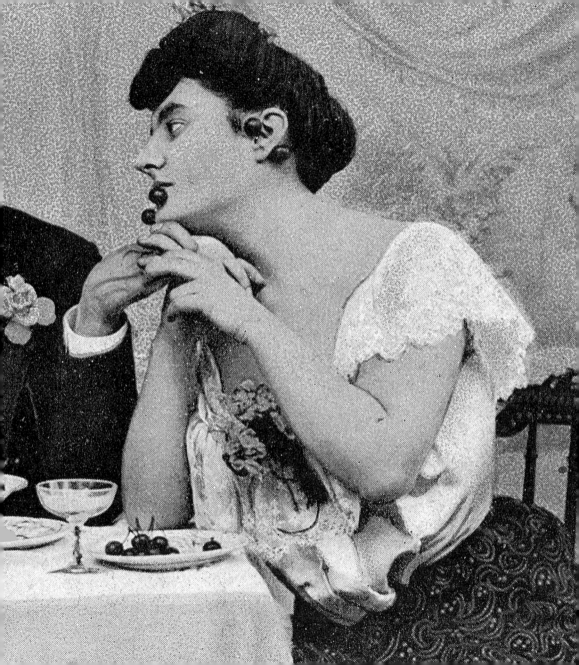

Beddy Bye

Across

1. "That's _____," Tom said, "half in Ernest."
6. All pigs have one.
9. A place where you can have a hot time.
10. Part of body that's short and wriggly.
11. Southern studly type (slang).
12. What they call someone who uses the rhythm method.
13. "_____ Strangelove" (abbrev.).
14. Bodily orifice.
15. The world's most popular game.
16. Primitive birth control device.
18. "Hey, baby, let's make a _____."
19. Something nice you call your wife.
20. Slightly inebriated.
21. Someone often found in bed with 13 across (abbrev.).
22. Cheap wine (slang).
24. "I've been _____."
25. Anger.
26. Something else that's quick as a bunny.
27. Adult playground.
28. One who plays.

Down

1. Give me all the _____ details.
2. "Please turn _____." Title of sexy British Movie.
3. Young, virginal society type.
4. "Turn me _____!"
5. Length of time elephant is pregnant.
6. What some people do to an ant (2 wds.).
7. What does the 2,000 pound canary weigh?
8. "Not _____, baby."
12. Another kind of piece (Latin).
14. Fishlike phallic symbol.
15. Kind of nuts.
16. Not as good as 27 across, but it'll do in a pinch.
17. What German couples get when they're not careful.
19. Popular show.
20. "If you don't like it, _____ it."
21. A good way to serve meat.
22. Eve was made from this.
23. One thing people dig for.
24. An outside adult playground.
26. Interjection.

Answers on page 272

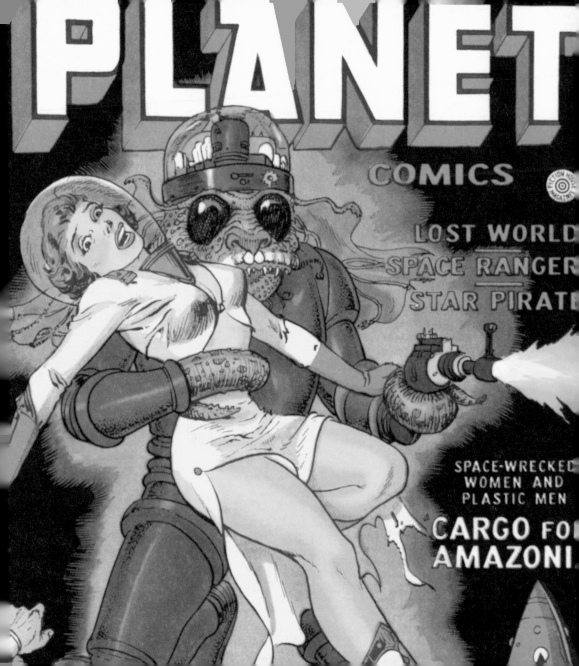

Funny Pages

Sometimes the comics are not just for kids—perhaps they never were. In the mid-1950s, the book Seduction of the Innocent by psychologist Fredrick Wertham argued that America's youth was being corrupted by comic book sex and violence. He thought that Wonder Woman's strength and independence showed her as a lesbian and that Batman and Robin, ". . . live in sumptuous quarters, with beautiful flowers in large vases, and have a butler . . . like a wish dream of two homosexuals living together." Out of this repression grew the Underground Comics Movement centered in hippie-central, 1960s San Francisco which explored all kinds of kinky taboos.

1954 Comics Code Highlights

- Profanity, obscenity, smut, vulgarity, or words or symbols which have acquired undesirable meanings are forbidden.

- Females shall be drawn realistically without exaggeration of any physical qualities.

- No comic magazine shall use the word horror or terror in its title.

- Nudity in any form is prohibited, as is indecent or undue exposure.

- Illicit sex relations are neither to be hinted at nor portrayed. Violent love scenes as well as sexual abnormalities are unacceptable.

WONDER WOMAN The feminist super hero was created in 1941 by William Marston who was inspired by his wife—who he considered the ideal liberated woman of her era—and Olive Byrne, who lived with the couple in a polyamorous relationship. Marston was known as an avid bondage enthusiast, an interest that was clearly reflected in early episodes that were full of bound women. Wonder Woman's indestructible bracelets, however, were not enough to protect her against the censorship brought about by the 1950s-era Comics Code Authority in reaction to allegations of a lesbian relationship with the Holiday girls. Before long she lost her outspoken feminism, and fell for Steve Trevor, Merman and even Birdman.

Funny Pages

LOST GIRLS (by Alan Moore and Melinda Gebbie; Top Shelf, 2006) An erotic graphic novel starring Alice (of Wonderland fame), Dorothy Gale (visitor to the land of Oz) and Wendy Darling (Peter Pan's muse) who meet as adults in a resort hotel in Austria and discuss their erotic pasts. "It seemed to us," Moore said in Science Fiction Weekly, "that sex, as a genre, was woefully under-represented in literature."

FRITZ THE CAT (by R. Crumb) Pioneer of 1960s underground comics movement in San Francisco, R. Crumb created the character Fritz the Cat who went on to star in the first X-rated full-length animated film. The box-office hit—about the misadventures of a frisky tomcat "who lives in a modern supercity of millions of animals"—was so hated by Crumb that he killed poor Fritz off in his comics with an icepick to the head.

BATMAN: THE DARK KNIGHT STRIKES AGAIN! (by Frank Miller; DC Comics, 2002) In this graphic novel several pages are devoted to the rough sex play between Superman and Wonder Woman, which— due to their super-human strength—causes earthquakes and tidal waves. "Where is the hero who threw me to the ground and took me as his rightful prize?" the Amazing Amazon cries.

TESTAMENT (by Douglas Rushkoff; Vertigo, 2006) This graphic novel series that takes place in the near future and simultaneously in biblical times does not shy away from depicting the sex and violence of either era. "Everybody thinks the Bible is boring and sanctimonious," Rushkoff said, "(but) the Bible is sexy . . . and violent."

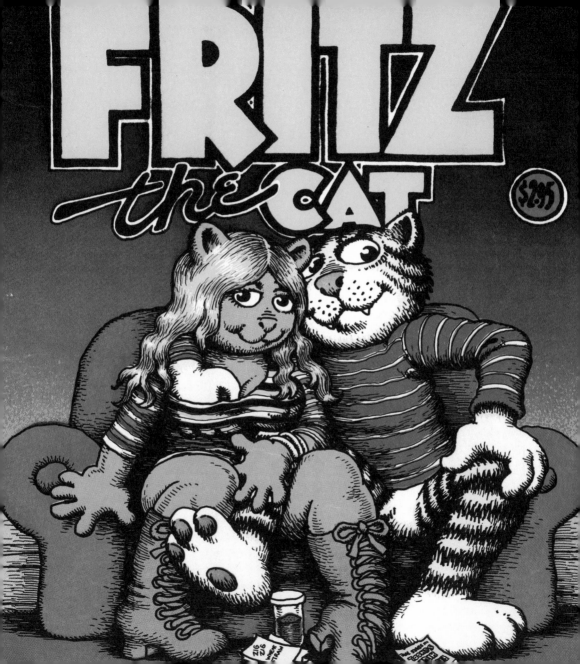

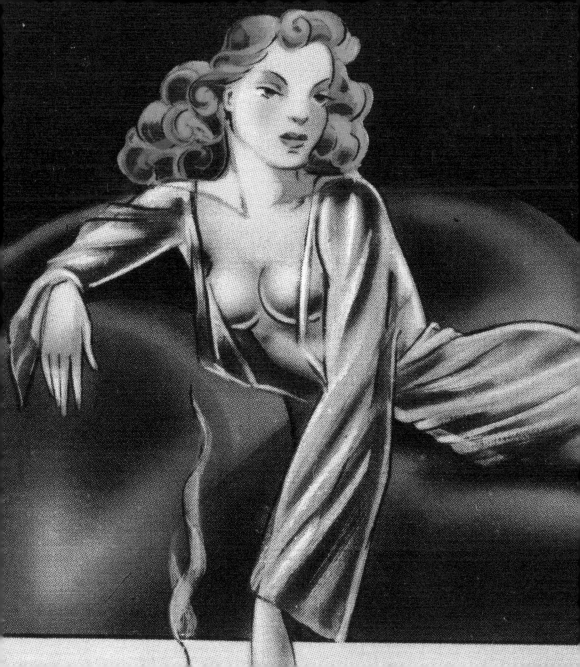

WHEN THE WEATHER IS HOT
I FEEL IN THE MOOD
TO TAKE OFF MY CLOTHES
AND RELAX IN THE NUDE!

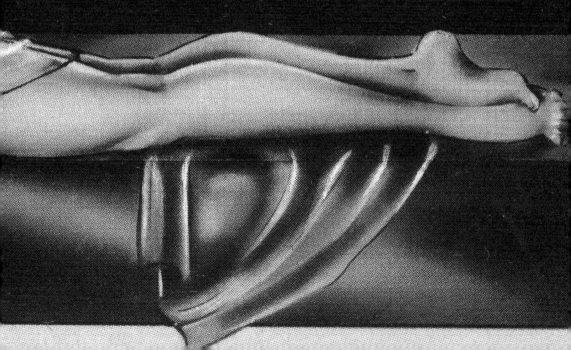

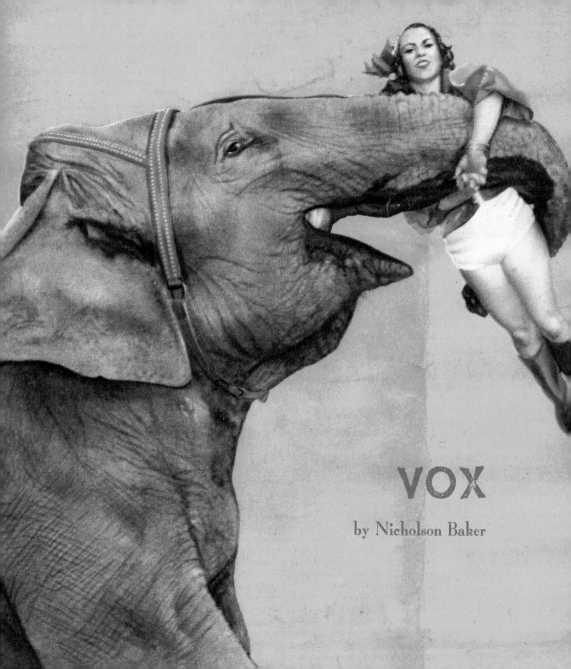

VOX

by Nicholson Baker

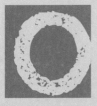oh, don't say that or I'll shoot."

"Hah hah! I like a man who knows what he likes. Do you want to hear what I thought about when I came in the shower yesterday?"

"By all means, tell me."

"Shall I tell you every nasty thing that comes into my head?"

"Yes."

"I will then," she said. "We went to the circus. It's funny, it excites me quite a bit just to tell you that I'm going to tell you. Doing that is probably the best part. It's just like that moment when you're lumbering around on the bed to get into opposite directions to do sixty-nine, that feeling of parting my legs over a man's face, *before* you put your hands on my back and pull me down, and my legs remember the feeling from the last time, the feeling of being locked into a preset position that is right for human bodies to be in, like putting a different lens on a camera, turning it until it clicks."

"And I," he said, "would feel the mattress change its slope, first on one side of my head, and then the other, as the weight of one of your knees and then the other pressed into it, and I'd look up at you and open my mouth and I'd slide my hands over your ass with my fingers splayed and hold your ass and pull you down to my tongue."

"Kha."

There was a pause.

"You there?" he asked.

"Yes."

"Tell me about the circus."

"Okay. Excuse me. I'm going to have to get a fresh towel pretty soon. This guy took me to the circus."

"The guy with the fancy stereo?"

"Another guy," she said. "it wasn't Ringling Brothers, it was some smaller-scale South American circus, with lots of elephants, and lots of women in spangles riding the elephants. It was incredibly hot in the tent, and everything had this reddish tint, because the sun was bright enough outside to make it through some of the tent seams, and I was wearing shorts and a T-shirt but I was soaked, and so was Lawrence, who was also wearing shorts and a T-shirt, and so was everyone around us, including the performers. There was some Venezuelan act in which a woman spun hard balls around very fast on long strings while two men played percussion behind her, and the balls smacked against the floorboards in interesting rhythms around her legs, and she was *streaming* with sweat, and quite beautiful, but in a way that I thought was vaguely like me, and suddenly the two men would stop hitting the drums and she would freeze and make this kind of trilling scream, a beautiful strange wild sound. She was just covered with sweat, she looked really wild, and the two man behind her were exceedingly good-looking, wearing wide-brimmed black hats with chin straps, and I momentarily wanted to be her, and while they were taking their bows I adapted my time-tested striptease fantasy, and I thought that I was this woman in the black spangles, and I was spinning these balls very fast, faster than she could, so they were a blur, so fast that somehow, like in a cartoon fight when it's just a blur from which things, pieces of clothing, fly outward, somehow my whole outfit was torn in pieces from my body, and flung out into the audience, so that when the drumming stopped and I froze suddenly and made my trilling scream, I was totally naked, and all these pieces of my costume were still floating aloft in all directions, and each man who caught some damp shred of costume was overpowered and took his place in line to fuck me, and the two percussionists played the drums the whole time, and then they stopped drumming and naturally they fucked me too. But that's just an aside. The elephant acts were what were interesting. I've ridden on an elephant once or twice in my life, when I was small, and I remember touching the big lobes of its head, and let me tell you, the skin is not smooth, it's warm and dry and quite bristly—that's how I remember it, anyway. And these were not little elephants, these were big old elephants, with big tusks. Well, these women were sliding down the side of the elephants, riding on the elephants heads, with their legs between the elephants' eyes, and repeatedly pivoting around on their bottoms on the elephants' backs, and they were wearing flesh-colored stockings, or tights, so it was not skin to skin, but even so, those little leotards are cut extremely high in the back, and I really started to be concerned about their bottoms, about whether they were more uncomfortable than their smiles let on, and I started thinking about whether if *I* were dressed in a very high-cut leotard I would like the sensation of the elephant's dry living skin on my bottom, and then, during the beginning of the very last big elephant promenade, one of the women was riding on the elephant's back with one leg in the air, and as the elephant turned I saw this woman's bottom, and even through the tights I could see that it was in fact red! She was the main elephant woman, I think. Anyhow, for the big finale she rode around on the elephant's tusks for a minute or two, sat on his trunk, fine fine, all gracefully executed but surprisingly suggestive, and then she did this thing that really shocked me. She took hold of one of the tusks and one of the ears, or somehow swung herself up, and then she lifted one of her knees so that it went right *into* the elephant's mouth, and she waited for a second for the elephant to clamp on to it, and then she threw her head back, and arched her back, and spread her arms wide, so she was held in the air supported entirely by her knee, which was stuffed in the elephant's mouth! I mean, think about the saliva! Think about those elephant molars that are gently but firmly taking hold of your upper calf and your mid-thigh, while this elephant tongue is there lounging with its giant taste-buds against your knee! The elephant did a full turn while she was swooning like this. Then she got down and took a bow and patted the elephant under his eye."

"Wow, that's better than *King Kong*." ∎

—From the novel written in 1992.

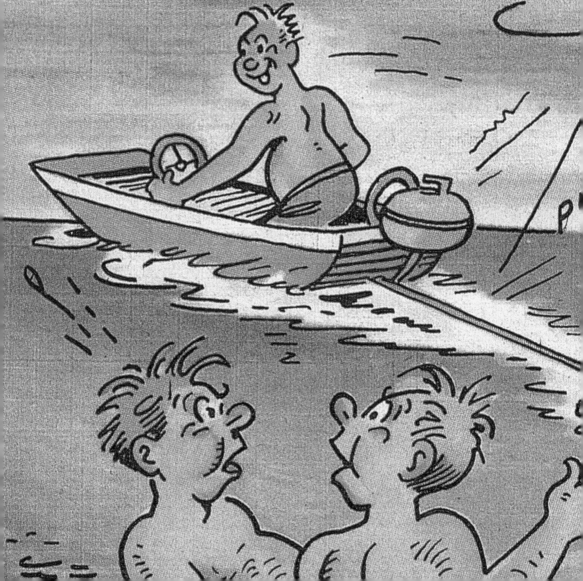

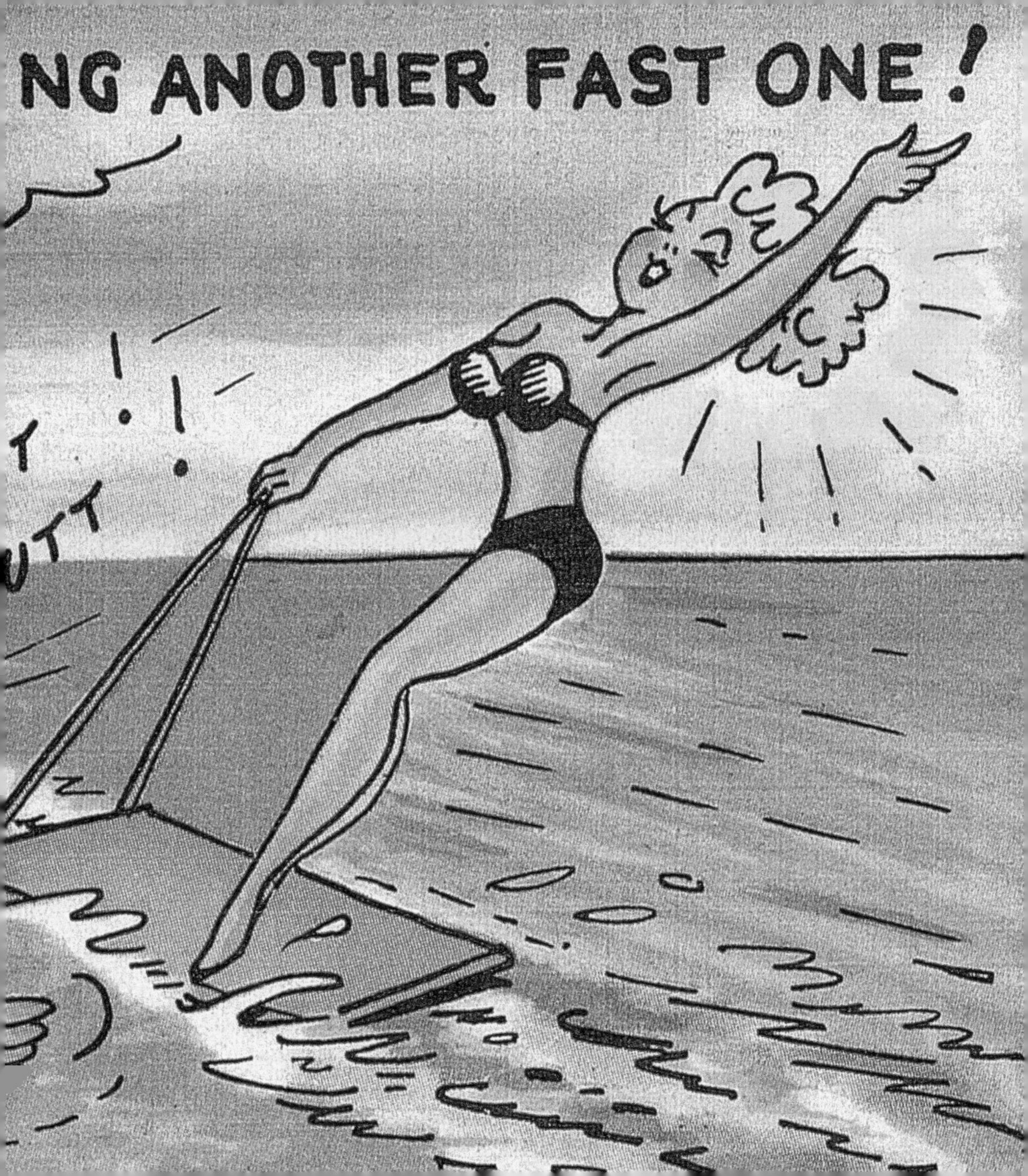
NG ANOTHER FAST ONE!
UTT

A Candle

John Suckling
c. 1630

There is a thing which in the light
Is seldom used, but in the night
It serves the maiden female crew,
The ladies, and the good-wives too.
They use to take it in their hand,
And then it will uprightly stand;
And to a hole they it apply,
Where by its goodwill it will die;
It spends, goes out, and still within
It leaves its moisture thick and thin.

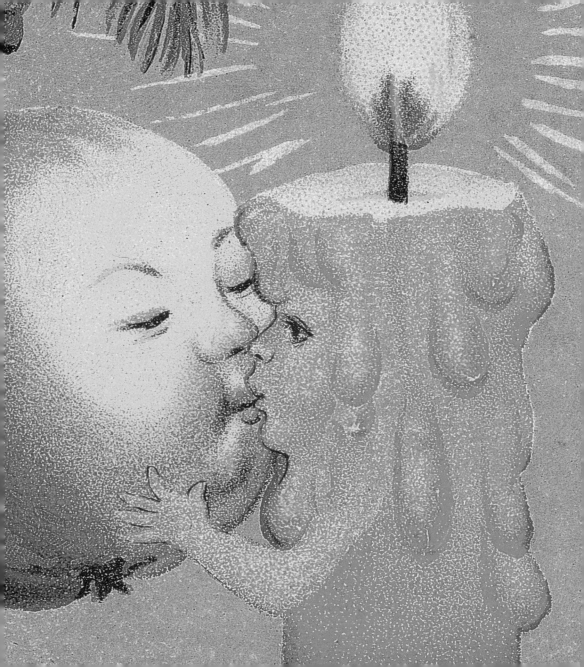

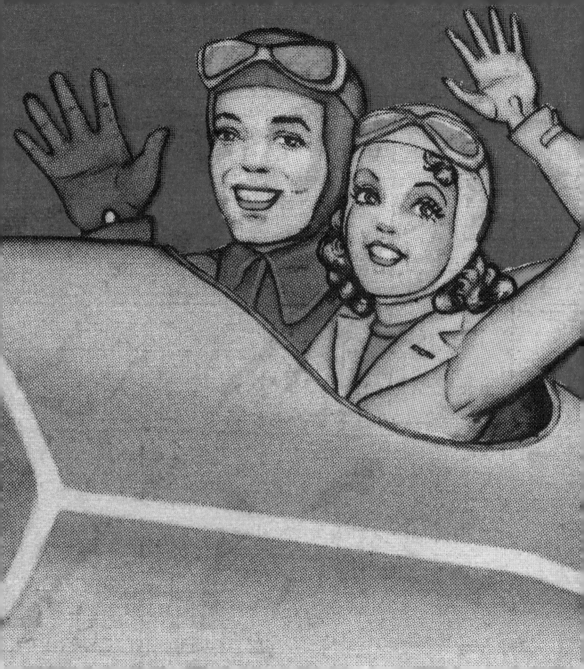

Mile High Club

The term "Mile High Club" refers to two people engaging in sexual activity (sexual intercourse) at an altitude of no less than 5,280 ft (a mile high above the earth) in an airplane.

Now, most veteran pilots will tell you that you need to be at the controls of an airplane in order to claim membership in this exclusive club. But over the years, the term Mile High Club has included those who make their mark in the lavatories aboard jetliners across the globe.

To spare the embarrassment for those who aren't quite daring enough to make their way back to the lav on a red-eye or transatlantic flight, mile high operations have been cropping up all over the country, offering couples the chance to climb aboard a custom-outfitted aircraft for their aerial pleasures.

—From *All About the Mile High Club*,
www.milehighclub.com

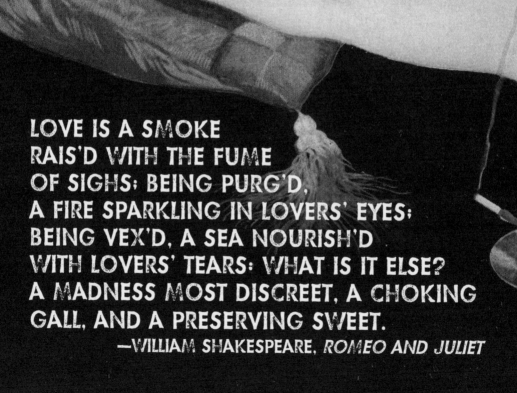

LOVE IS A SMOKE
RAIS'D WITH THE FUME
OF SIGHS; BEING PURG'D,
A FIRE SPARKLING IN LOVERS' EYES;
BEING VEX'D, A SEA NOURISH'D
WITH LOVERS' TEARS: WHAT IS IT ELSE?
A MADNESS MOST DISCREET, A CHOKING
GALL, AND A PRESERVING SWEET.
                —WILLIAM SHAKESPEARE, *ROMEO AND JULIET*